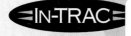

ctive

s

Pavilion

Developing and Supporting Effective Staff Supervision: A reader to support the delivery of staff supervision training for those working with vulnerable children, adults and their families

© Jane Wonnacott

Published by:
Pavilion Publishing and Media Ltd
Rayford House, School Road,
Hove, BN3 5HX
Tel: 01273 434943
Fax: 01273 227308
Email: info@pavpub.com
Web: www.pavpub.com

Published 2014.

Reader ISBN: 978-1-908993-55-7
Suite ISBN: 978-1-909810-34-1
epdf ISBN: 978-1-909810-39-6
epub ISBN: 978-1-909810-41-9
MOBI ISBN: 978-1-909810-40-2

Pavilion is the leading publisher and provider of professional development products and services for workers in the health, social care, education and community safety sectors. We believe that everyone has the right to fulfil their potential and we strive to supply products and services that help raise standards, promote best practices and support continuing professional development.

Author: Jane Wonnacott
Production editor: Catherine Ansell-Jones, Pavilion Publishing and Media Ltd
Cover design: Emma Dawe, Pavilion Publishing and Media Ltd
Page layout and typesetting: Phil Morash, Pavilion Publishing and Media Ltd
Printing: CMP Digital Print Solutions

Contents

Preface

In 2005 the revised, third edition of *Staff Supervision in Social Care* by Tony Morrison was published. The resource has inspired and continues to inspire many supervisors from a wide range of professions, stretching their thinking, developing their skills and giving them confidence in their role within the ever-changing social care environment.

In 2008 Tony Morrison and In-Trac Training & Consultancy were commissioned by the Children's Workforce Development Council to deliver a national training programme for the supervisors of newly qualified social workers. During this process the materials in *Staff Supervision in Social Care* (2001; 2005) were revisited and at times amended or developed, taking account of training materials that Tony Morrison, Jane Wonnacott and members of the In-Trac team had been using in their training courses.

While this reader aims to draw out the main building blocks of the supervision model outlined in *Staff Supervision in Social Care* (2001; 2005), as well as the more recent developments to the approach, it is not meant to be a 'dumbing down' or an oversimplification of the issues. The underpinning belief throughout is that working with human relationships is complex and demanding and cannot be packaged neatly into a one-size-fits-all prescribed way of responding. The supervision model and accompanying tools have always been designed to enable practitioners to respond to the individual nature of the issues they are working with and create a reflective space for exploring challenging issues and ideas, using the knowledge generated through the process to inform both frontline practice and the strategic direction of the organisation.

The joy of Morrison's approach has always been the way in which it takes complex ideas, makes them accessible to a wide audience and alongside this gives people tools to help them in their day-to-day practice. This publication aims to continue this approach by reminding readers of core aspects of the model which, if implemented, will provide the foundations for an approach to supervision that makes a real difference to those using social care and health services.

Acknowledgements

This reader and accompanying training pack would not have been possible without the work and wisdom of Tony Morrison. In-Trac were privileged to work closely with Tony and were inspired by his enthusiasm for both the importance of good, high quality training and the crucial role that supervision plays in health and social care organisations. Tony was never one for standing still and I hope that the reader and training pack do justice to Tony's past work, demonstrate its continued relevance and take it forward with some new developments and ideas.

Many thanks to the In-Trac associate team for their work in delivering numerous supervision training events and in keeping the materials alive through constantly thinking about how to adapt them in our ever-changing environment.

I am particularly grateful to Jacquie Morrison for supporting the publication of Tony's material and to Pavilion Publishing and Media for the opportunity to put into the public domain training materials that have not formerly been available.

Introduction

This publication has a dual purpose. Firstly, it has been written to provide background reading for trainers delivering supervision training programmes derived from the accompanying training pack *Developing and Supporting Effective Staff Supervision* (2013). In this role it provides background reading for trainers delivering the programme, which will help in using the PowerPoint slides, explaining the rationale for the exercises and handling group discussions. It might also be useful as additional reading material for participants.

Secondly, the reader is designed to be a standalone publication summarising the core elements of Tony Morrison's supervision model outlined in *Staff Supervision in Social Care* (2001; 2005) and making this accessible to the widest possible audience. In this role it also brings into the public domain developments of the model that Tony had been working on with Jane Wonnacott and In-Trac Training and Consultancy prior to his death in 2010. It should be stressed that this reader does not replace Tony Morrison's original work; it simply sets out to extract those aspects of the model which must be at the heart of any training programme and are non-negotiable if the integrity of the model is to be maintained.

The reader should therefore be of interest to anyone who works in health or social care and has a role as either a supervisor or a supervisee. The terms 'health' and 'social care' are used in their widest possible sense and include statutory, voluntary and private organisations providing community, residential and day care services for adults and/or children and their families. It is the premise of the reader that the principles of good supervision practice can be applied in a variety of settings, although each organisation will have different challenges as to how best to manage the practical arrangements necessary for effective delivery.

Supervision in health and social care – the current context

The role of supervision within the helping professions has a long history and this is particularly the case within social work and therapeutic services. Approaches have, however, varied from the psychodynamic to a focus on task completion/compliance and not all organisations have consistently prioritised supervision as a key part of the service. Concerns about the quality of service delivery across a wide range of services including social work (Social Work Task Force/Social Work Reform Board), learning disability residential care (eg. Department of Health's Winterbourne Review (2012)), residential child care (eg. Waterhouse Inquiry in 2000), and early years (Plymouth Safeguarding Children Board (2010)) have brought the importance of good quality supervision to the fore and there is accumulating practice evidence of the very real difference that supervision can make. Empirical research is lagging behind practice knowledge but a review of the research evidence (Carpenter *et al*, 2012) concluded that good supervision is associated with:

- job satisfaction
- commitment to the organisation
- staff retention
- employees' perceptions of the support they receive from the organisation.

There is now a general acceptance that supervision is an important aspect of organisational life, with the Social Work Reform Board's standard for employers stating that:

'Supervision provides a safe environment for critical reflection, challenge and professional support that operates alongside an organisation's appraisal process. It includes time for reflection on practice issues that arise in the course of everyday work and can help social workers and their managers to do their jobs more effectively. It enables social workers to develop their capacity to use their experiences to review practice, receive feedback on their performance, build emotional resilience and think reflectively about the relationships they have formed with children, adults and families.' (Social Work Reform Board, 2012)

A belief in the importance of supervision for all those working in the human services was the driver for the work of Tony Morrison in the first edition of *Staff Supervision in Social Care* (2001) and similarly this reader is underpinned by the following assumptions.

- **Supervision is part of the intervention with services' users**.
  It is not an 'add on' but inextricably linked to the experience of adults, children and families who are receiving services from health and social care staff.

- **Good supervision makes more difference than we will ever know**. The impact of supervision is hard to measure, as evidenced by the lack of empirical research; it is likely, however, that the effect of good supervision is far reaching and that supervisors frequently have much greater influence on staff and practice than they may imagine.

- **Supervision is the basis for practice leadership**. The role of the supervisor as an experienced professional with the professional authority to both support and develop practice is key. For example, research carried out by SCIE in adult social care (Lambley & Marrable, 2013) noted that supervisees valued supervisors who were from the same profession as them, were up-to-date with the latest theory and practice, and were therefore able to support frontline practice.

- **Early experiences of supervision have a powerful impact on professional confidence, competence, identity and direction**. Supervisors of staff in the early stages of their career have a unique opportunity to influence the values, professionalism, practice and confidence of the worker.

These beliefs are in line with a drive across the human services sector to establish supervision as a core activity supporting good practice. However, despite this, evidence suggests that many organisations may struggle to embed and sustain effective supervision. Requirements for supervision in early years settings in the Early Years Foundation Stage (Department for Education, 2012) may seem too daunting and difficult to implement; residential care settings similarly may be put off by the complexity of establishing supervision sessions in a shift system; and even where there is a long history of supervision in professions such as social work, there is evidence that high quality supervision is not always being delivered consistently (Community Care, 2013). Perhaps the task in many organisations seems too large when faced with limited resources? It is not uncommon to hear that although there is a will to deliver good supervision, it is seen as too difficult or too time consuming or too costly. However, the costs of not establishing a culture of effective supervision are also great and this reader aims to refocus on the fundamental aspects of an effective supervision model that is most likely to make a real difference to the quality of services delivered to adults, children and their families.

The core components of this supervision model

This model of supervision has become colloquially known as the 4x4x4 model since it recognises the interrelationship between the four key functions of supervision, the impact of the quality of supervision on four key stakeholders and the use of the four stages of the supervision cycle to deliver reflective supervision. The importance of this is that the model moves beyond a static focus on functions to a dynamic, integrated approach which recognises the central importance of effective supervision across the whole system.

The elements of the 4x4x4 model and how we might define reflective supervision are explored further in Chapter 2. Central to the success of the model are number of core components, which need to be the focus of any supervision training programme.

Recognition that supervision makes a difference to outcomes for service users

This approach to supervision has at its heart a recognition that supervision is much more than a 'nice to have' added extra; it has a fundamental effect on the way staff feel about their work, their behaviour towards service users and colleagues, and their knowledge and skills. As a result, supervision has a corresponding impact on the experience of service users and ultimately outcomes for adults, children and their families. The underpinning research and theory relating to the link between the quality of supervision and outcomes for service users are explored further in Chapter 1.

The importance of the supervisory relationship

Recent work focusing on relationship-based practice (Ruch, 2010) has identified the key role that emotions and relationships play in our work with service users. This approach to supervision recognises the centrality of relationships and the importance of developing a positive relationship between the supervisor and the supervisee, which is then mirrored in the way that the supervisee works with service users. This is explored further in Chapter 3.

The role of the supervision agreement as a foundation for the relationship

Since a positive supervisory relationship is at the heart of this approach to supervision, attention needs to be paid to making sure that this is on a firm footing, that supervision is a safe place where boundaries are clear and that the supervisee is able to explore their practice openly and honestly. Too often supervision contracts or agreements are documents prescribed by the organisation which are the same for every supervisee and fail to take account of the individual nature of each supervisory relationship. Central to this model is the need to pay attention to all the factors that might impact on the relationship and to make sure that these are 'on the table' rather than 'under the table' where they could unintentionally inhibit an open and honest exploration of relevant issues. The role of the agreement in promoting this approach is explored in Chapter 3 and its positive impact on working to improve performance is considered in Chapter 7.

The interrelationship between feelings, thoughts and action

Gibbs (2001), in presenting a case for re-focusing supervision to one which was most likely to retain staff, argued for an approach that enabled a focus on the impact of feelings and thoughts on action and perception. Such an approach involves working with emotions, valuing intuitive responses and combining these with analytical thinking in order to inform judgements, decisions and plans. This approach is at the heart of the 4x4x4 model and is explored throughout the reader, but particularly in Chapters 3 and 4.

The role of the supervision cycle in promoting reflective practice, critical thinking and defensible (recorded) decision making

At the heart of this approach is the supervision cycle. Based on Kolb's (1988) adult learning cycle, it encourages supervisors to ask questions which move beyond task completion to understanding the interrelationship between feelings, thoughts and actions. As such, the model allows for an approach which recognises that often in the human services decisions are based on professional judgement and are finely balanced. An important aspect of good practice is being able to explain the reasons for decisions to service users and colleagues in order to foster transparency and appropriate debate and challenge. Recording the reasons for decisions becomes easier when supervision has allowed space for the critical reflection and critical thinking underpinning the work to take place.

Defining supervision

The definition of supervision used in this reader is the definition developed by Morrison and set out in *Staff Supervision in Social Care* (2001).

'Supervision is a process by which one worker is given responsibility by the organisation to work with another worker(s) in order to meet certain organisational, professional and personal objectives, which together promote the best outcomes for service users.
These objectives and functions are:
1. Competent accountable performance (managerial function)
2. Continuing professional development (developmental / formative function)
3. Personal support (supportive / restorative function)
4. Engaging the individual with the organisation (mediation function).'

Although at first sight this definition may seem to simply set out the functions of supervision, it does, in fact, establish that:

- it is more than an event or 'session' but is a process, based on a set of relationships mandated by the organisation

- whatever the supervisor's role in relation to the supervisee, supervision is an authority relationship

- it is a complex set of activities which are interrelated but could be delivered by one or more people acting in different roles.

It is important to be clear about what supervision is not. Supervision is not the same as mentoring, coaching or consultation, although similar skills may be used. Morrison (2005) distinguished between these activities as follows.

Consultation
'A structured negotiated process involving two or more staff in which the consultant is identified as having some expertise which is used to facilitate a developmental or problem-solving process.' (Morrison, 1998)

Mentoring

'A mentor is the person who helps another learn from their experience in the workplace. It is a developmental alliance between equals.' (Hay, 1995)

Coaching

'A coach is an individual who helps another identify and remedy performance or skill deficit via modelling and rehearsal.' (Hay, 1995)

Thus the supervisor may help their supervisee learn or develop using similar skills to the mentor or coach and a supervisee may consult with their supervisor, but these interactions are only part of the supervisor's role, which encompasses an overall responsibility for the supervisee's practice, welfare and development.

Delivering supervision

How this model of supervision is delivered will depend upon the nature of the organisation and roles and responsibilities within it. This reader and the training pack focus on the one-to-one relationship with a supervisor, which will be the basis of both formal and informal (ad hoc) discussions. Formal planned one-to-one sessions are at the heart of the approach and one practice enquiry found that this was the preferred form of supervision for the majority of supervisees (Lambley & Marrable, 2013). However, relationships are not confined to specific time slots and there will be times when ad hoc discussions are an important part of the process. No one way of supervising is perfect but what is crucial is that supervisors have an awareness of the advantages and disadvantages of the different approaches. Morrison (2005) sets out a framework for thinking about the interface between formal/informal/planned/ad hoc supervision.

Figure 1.0: Structures for supervision

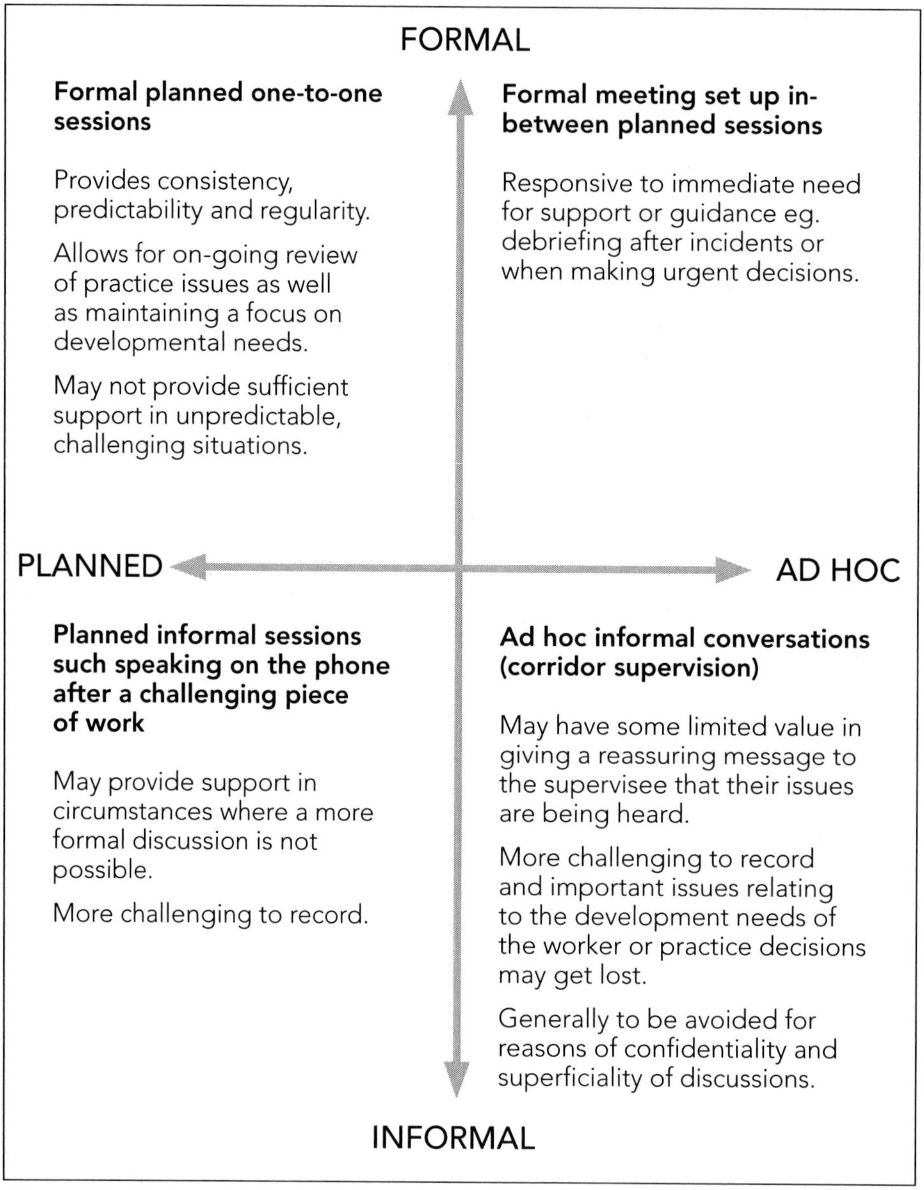

	FORMAL	
Formal planned one-to-one sessions Provides consistency, predictability and regularity. Allows for on-going review of practice issues as well as maintaining a focus on developmental needs. May not provide sufficient support in unpredictable, challenging situations.		**Formal meeting set up in-between planned sessions** Responsive to immediate need for support or guidance eg. debriefing after incidents or when making urgent decisions.
PLANNED		**AD HOC**
Planned informal sessions such speaking on the phone after a challenging piece of work May provide support in circumstances where a more formal discussion is not possible. More challenging to record.		**Ad hoc informal conversations (corridor supervision)** May have some limited value in giving a reassuring message to the supervisee that their issues are being heard. More challenging to record and important issues relating to the development needs of the worker or practice decisions may get lost. Generally to be avoided for reasons of confidentiality and superficiality of discussions.
	INFORMAL	

In some settings, as well as the methods above, aspects of supervision may be delivered by an additional supervisor, or a supervisor may provide supplementary supervision to a group of their supervisees. Chapter 2 explores some of the issues relating to the delivery of the model where such arrangements occur.

References

Carpenter J, Webb C, Bostock L & Coomber C (2012) *Effective Supervision in Social Work and Social Care*. London: SCIE.

Community Care (2013) *Third of UK's social workers not currently receiving supervision* [online]. Available at: http://www.communitycare.co.uk/2013/06/18/third-of-uks-social-workers-not-currently-receiving-supervision/ (accessed November 2013).

Department for Education (2012) *Statutory Framework for Early Years Foundation Stage* [online]. Available at: http://www.education.gov.uk/aboutdfe/statutory/g00213120/eyfs-statutory-framework (accessed November 2013).

Department of Health (2012) *Transforming Care: A national response to Winterbourne View Hospital*. London: DH.

Gibbs JA (2001) Maintaining frontline workers in child protection: a case for re-focusing supervision. *Child Abuse Review* **10** 323–335.

Hay J (1995) *Transformational Mentoring: Creating development alliances for changing organizational cultures*. New York: McGraw-Hill.

Kolb D (1988) *Experience as a Source of Learning and Development*. London: Prentice Hall.

Lambley S & Marrable T (2013) *Practice Enquiry into Supervision in a Variety of Adult Care Settings Where There are Health and Social Care Practitioners Working Together* (pp. 15). London: SCIE.

Morrison T (1998) *Casework Consultation: A practical guide for consultation to work with sex offenders and other high risk clients*. London: Whiting and Birch.

Morrison T (2001) *Staff Supervision in Social Care*. Brighton: Pavilion.

Morrison T (2005) *Staff Supervision in Social Care* (3rd edition). Brighton: Pavilion.

Plymouth Safeguarding Children Board (2010) *Serious Case Review for Nursery Z*. Plymouth: Plymouth Safeguarding Children Board.

Ruch G (2010) The contemporary context of relationship-based practice. In: G Ruch, D Turney & A Ward (eds) *Relationship Based Social Work*. London: JKP.

Social Work Reform Board (2012) *Standards for Employers of Social Workers in England and Supervision Framework 2012*. Available at: http://media.education.gov.uk/assets/files/pdf/standards%20for%20employers.pdf (accessed November 2013).

Chapter 1: What difference can supervision make?

Supervision is only useful if it makes a real difference to the quality of service delivery and has a positive impact on the lives of users of health and social care services. Unfortunately, however, the research base in relation to the impact of supervision on outcomes for service users is limited.

Carpenter *et al*'s (2012) review of the empirical research concluded that the evidence base is limited and that further research is required. However, despite the paucity of empirical research the study did conclude that good supervision is associated with:

- job satisfaction
- commitment to the organisation
- staff retention
- employees' perceptions of the support they receive from the organisation.

Since retaining staff is important for organisations and children and families alike, on this measure alone it is clear that providing 'good' supervision is something that is important to pay attention to.

Evidence from practice, particularly in the field of child protection, has pointed to the difference that supervision can make. For example, studies of serious case reviews have noted:

'Practitioners who are well supported, receive supervision and have access to training are more likely to think clearly and exercise professional discretion.' (Brandon *et al*, 2005)

'Effective and accessible supervision is essential if staff are to be helped to put in practice the critical thinking required ... it needs to help practitioners to think, to explain, to understand ... it is essential to help practitioners cope with the emotional demands of the job.' (Brandon *et al*, 2008)

Within an early years environment, a serious case review into the abuse of children in a nursery setting commented:

'This review has identified the urgent need to develop effective staff supervision within early years settings. With no formal structures allowing staff to reflect on their own work and practice within the nursery, there was no opportunity for any discomfort with K's increasing sexualised behaviour to be aired. Lack of supervision also meant there was no effective means to manage performance and challenge inappropriate behaviour such as use of mobile phones within the nursery.' (Plymouth Safeguarding Children Board, 2010, p.34)

A small, unpublished study into the impact of supervision on outcomes for children found that the style of the supervisor is an important factor (Wonnacott, 2004). Thirteen social work supervisors and 14 practitioners were interviewed about their experiences of supervision. This was followed by a case file analysis to track the impact of supervision on 12 of the cases over a five-month period. Three types of supervision process were identified.

1. Active intrusive

This was the most common type, where the supervisor adopted a very direct approach to make sure the social worker carried out key tasks. Its benefit was that the supervisor had a good knowledge of the social worker's cases and could ensure that their work was done in accordance with organisational procedures. However, little attention was paid to the worker's feelings, or to worker–user relations.

2. Active reflexive

These supervisors were active and knew about the work being undertaken, but engaged supervisees in a collaborative and reflective process. Attention was paid to the social worker's feelings and to the social worker–user dynamic as an additional source of information. When the social worker was struggling or had lost focus, these supervisors helped them reflect on what was going on, using challenging and user-focused questions. This included the supervisor observing the social worker's relationship with the family to gain an accurate assessment of the social workers' strengths and limitations.

3. Passive avoidant

This was a relationship where the supervisor regarded the practitioner as being competent, and left it up to him/her to decide if and when contact with the supervisor was required. Although this left the social worker in control at one level, the supervisor effectively abandoned him/her, and therefore the employer was unable to take responsibility for their work. If things went wrong, the social worker, supervisor, users and employer were all vulnerable.

Table 1.1: Comparing three types of supervisor styles

Active intrusive	Active reflexive	Passive avoidant
Prescriptive	Collaborative	Laissez-faire
Knows the cases	Knows the cases	Cases not known
Task and procedure	Task and process	Supervisee-led
Assessment of supervisees and output	Overall assessment of supervisee's competence	Lack of assessment
Checking up	Reflection and challenge	Avoidant
Directive	Developmental focus including emotional competence	Collusive

Wonnacott (2004)

In summary, the strongest links between supervision and good outcomes were when the supervisor had an accurate assessment of the social worker's knowledge and skills, and had the capacity to develop an effective relationship within which there could be an open, honest exploration of practice. Emotionally intelligent supervisory practice is important here, and it is explored further in Chapter 4.

Despite the relative lack of empirical research into supervisory practice there is consistent evidence about what service users find most helpful in their relationships with the helping professions and what appears to work most effectively in promoting good outcomes. These studies can inform our understanding of what might work best in supervisory practice, since the role of the supervisor will be to promote such practice and model in their own supervisory style the behaviours that they are wishing to promote.

One example of a meta-analysis of what succeeds in promoting effective outcomes is a major review of what works in family support services for vulnerable children carried out for the Irish Government (McKeown, 2000), which found that four main factors accounted for change. These were:

- 40% characteristics of the user (IQ, history, socio-economic status and social support)

- 30% worker relationship with the user, especially empathy, goal setting and planning

- 15% method of intervention, for example, family therapy or parental education

- 15% degree of hope verbally expressed by the user about change, for example, 'This time I will kick my drugs habit'.

Hence the combination of a really good assessment, which sought to understand the characteristics and situation of the user, combined with establishing an empathic and structured relationship, accounted for 70% of the change effort. Only after a clear assessment has been undertaken does choice of method become significant. Verbal expression of hope is also seen to play a very modest role – a factor that less-experienced staff may miss.

This suggests that the two most important areas for the supervisor to focus on are:

- the capacity of the worker to understand the service users they are working with and therefore assess accurately how best to work with them to meet their needs

- the worker's ability to establish and maintain effective relationships with service users.

The challenge for supervisors is to consider how their supervisory style can most effectively achieve these goals. What type of conversations with supervisees will really get to the heart of their understanding of the service user? How might the quality of the supervisory relationship affect what is shared in supervision and hence inform the supervisor's understanding of the relationship between the supervisee and the service users they are working with? The model of supervision outlined within this reader and explored fully in Chapter 2 is designed to support a style of supervision which is most likely to achieve these goals.

The figure below develops further an understanding of the link between supervision and outcomes for service users. It explores the interrelationship between a clarity of purpose within supervision, the ability to engage with emotions both within supervision and with service users, and the impact this has on the worker's observational skills, as well as the way they use this within their relationships. Where these factors are working together positively, assessments are likely to be more accurate and plans most effective.

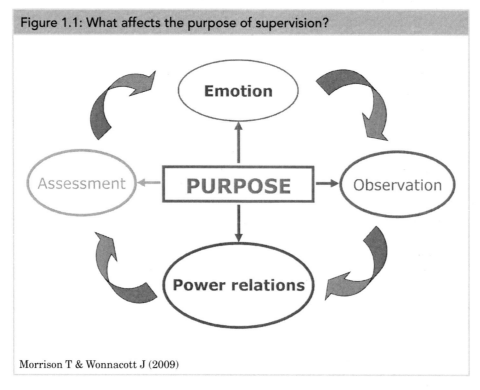

Figure 1.1: What affects the purpose of supervision?

Morrison T & Wonnacott J (2009)

For example, if during the development of the supervisory relationship it has been made explicit that supervision is a place to explore fears, feelings, uncertainties and mistakes, the supervisee will be more likely to talk about relationships with service users that are worrying them. This may, for example, involve fear of violence and the worker may be aware that they are avoiding visiting a family home. When they have not felt able to explore this in supervision they will be more likely to protect themselves through further avoidant behaviour, 'not seeing' and therefore not challenging any risky behaviours. They may allow powerful family members to dominate and consequently fail to assess accurately the needs of vulnerable children and/or adults. Conversely, the worker who has explored their fears and worries about their practice is more likely to understand the origins of their fears (which may or may not be accurate) and develop strategies for managing the task (for example, co-working). In this situation the appropriate use of power and authority is more likely, enabling an accurate assessment of the needs of all involved.

The collaborative supervision cycle

All the evidence explored so far in this chapter points towards a collaborative supervision cycle in which supervision reinforces good practice, which in turn reinforces good supervision.

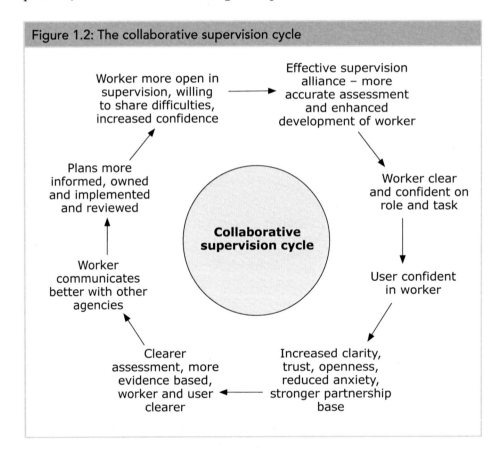

Figure 1.2: The collaborative supervision cycle

This can be contrasted with the compromised supervision cycle in which poor supervision or lack of supervision reinforces poor practice.

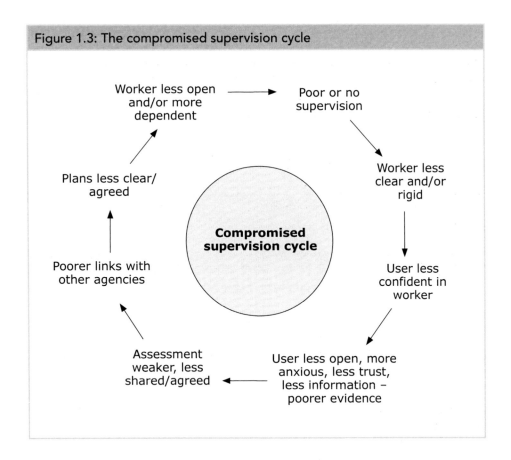

Figure 1.3: The compromised supervision cycle

Both cycles show that clarity and confidence have a powerful impact on the quality of the worker's relationship with the user, as well as on their observation and assessment of the user's situation. These core processes affect two further processes: the worker's communication with other agencies, and the user's engagement in the planning process. Underlying these cycles are the powerful connections that exist between clarity, power, engagement, communication, planning and reflection. Where these are aligned with others in a committed and shared purpose, people can discover new skills and confidence.

It is now possible to begin to build a model for effective supervision. This was originally described as involving six stages (Morrison, 2005) but was later developed in Morrison's training materials to seven stages, with the inclusion of coaching as one of the elements.

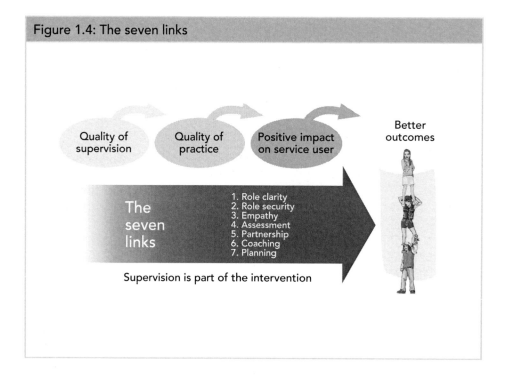

Figure 1.4: The seven links

The seven links

1. Role clarity

This starts with the supervisor being clear about his/her role and the mandate that they have from their organisation, as well as understanding what good supervision looks like and any expectations set out within a supervision policy. For the practitioner, supervision provides the opportunity to clarify their role and responsibility, or to re-focus when there has been confusion or conflict over their role. For example, for a newly qualified member of staff the transition from their previous student role and identity to their new role is a major task. Hence in these circumstances it is very important that the supervisor is clear about what is and what is not expected of the worker and how supervision can be used to support them in their practice. In turn, the practitioner needs to be clear about their role with the user and to help the user to clarify their role in working with the service provider.

2. Role security

Practitioners need not only to be clear about their role but also feel secure in it. Role security comes from a combination of knowledge, skills, experience and support. For any member of staff who lacks experience in their role, it is essential that anxieties and doubts can be raised and resolved, providing a secure base from which they can practice effectively. It is important to recognise that even experienced members of staff, if taking on new responsibilities, may lack confidence and a sense of security. Role security also depends on the supervisee being given an appropriate workload at the appropriate level. In turn, the worker's clarity, composure, knowledge and responsiveness enable service users to develop confidence and trust in the practitioner.

3. Emotional competence and empathy

The supervisor's empathy and emotional capacity create a secure and collaborative working relationship. This allows the supervisee to develop sufficient trust to be open about their doubts, feelings and mistakes, as well as to take risks, accept new challenges and take the initiative. In turn, the practitioner's empathy and understanding enable vulnerable and anxious service users to be open about their needs and reveal the real nature of their concerns. Empathy helps the user to talk about emotional issues – for instance, experiences of loss or trauma – or moral issues, such as a drinking problem or a parent's approach to boundaries and sanctions for their children.

4. Accurate observation and assessment

The three previous elements establish the clarity, security and collaborative approach in which the supervisor can make and share an accurate assessment of the worker's knowledge and skills. This is the basis for the future development of the worker through supervision; if this hasn't been established, the worker cannot be open with the supervisor and the supervisor's assessment is unlikely to be accurate. In turn, the practitioner who can explain the purpose and process of their work clearly and engage openly with the service user will create a more accurate assessment of need. In addition, this approach to assessment is much more likely to lead to the resulting plans being shared between colleagues.

5. Partnership and power

The clarity of the supervisor's role, collaborative approach and accurate assessment of the worker is most likely to result in an appropriate use of authority which is neither collusive nor punitive. Clarity of role will give the supervisee confidence to engage in an open, honest debate with the supervisor and for each party to feel comfortable in challenging the other. An important aspect of this is the capacity to work effectively with diversity within the supervisory relationship and for power and authority not to be over- or under-used on account of factors such as race, gender, sexual orientation etc. In turn, the practitioner will be clear with the service user about their authority and its limits, and will be able to establish a suitable level of partnership reflecting their assessment of the needs, strengths and risks in the case.

6. Coaching

The supervisor plays a key role in developing the worker's practice skills. This occurs through a combination of modelling, practice observation, feedback, reflection, problem solving and knowledge enhancement. However, practice skills are developed not only through the supervisor but also through the modelling, mentoring, shadowing, co-working and feedback that occurs in a healthy and collaborative team setting. The skill for the supervisor lies in creating the opportunities for these peer-practice learning situations while helping the practitioner to identify what they are learning from these experiences. In the same way, the worker has to build the user's skills, strengths and coping capacities through practical problem-solving work. At times the worker may act as a coach, using observation, providing feedback, practical advice, teaching strategies and other techniques to grow their skills.

7. Planning

The final link is planning. The supervisor can only develop timely and appropriate supervision plans if they are based on the earlier stages. In turn, the practitioner uses supervision as a place to analyse the needs, strengths and risks of their cases, and to identify priorities and plans to address these issues. The worker can then involve service users in developing plans, and in monitoring and reviewing their progress towards agreed goals that improve their lives.

Does supervision make a difference?

In summary, this chapter argues that there is ample evidence from practice that a style of supervision which challenges and supports staff to think and practice creatively will make a very real difference to the quality of practice and outcomes for service users. The foundation for this must be the development of an open and honest relationship with a supervisor where fears and anxieties can be explored and the quality of practice evaluated.

A rough look at the costs and potential benefits of supervision sets out a compelling case for seeing supervision as a necessity – not a luxury.

Table 1.2: Costs and benefits of effective supervision

Costs	Benefits
■ Staff time	■ Job satisfaction
■ Staff training	■ Commitment to the organisation
■ Support for supervisors	■ Staff retention
■ Physical space	■ Reduced stress/sickness through staff feeling supported
	■ Consistent relationships with service users
	■ Creative thinking
	■ Recognition of the emotional impact of the work and the way this may affect decision making
	■ Risk sensible practice and defensible decision making

We cannot therefore afford not to supervise effectively. When we are struggling with scarce resources and dealing with ever more complex problems, we need to foster resilience by providing frontline staff with the scaffolding they need to work with the most vulnerable members of our society with the emotional intelligence and compassion that will make a difference. Relationships are at the heart of good practice and relationships must be at the heart of the way we supervise and manage as well. The model of supervision described within this reader is designed to support this approach to supervision.

In preparation for the delivery of a training programme for social work supervisors, Tony Morrison wrote.

'It would be hard to overstate the importance of good supervision at a time when there is such intense political and professional concern about the quality of children's services. It is in such a climate that the role of supervision in leading practice as well as managing performance is so critical. Good supervision and good outcomes for children and families are inextricably bound together. Ensuring that all those responsible for the supervision of staff are properly trained and supported must therefore rank as one of the most urgent priorities within any children and young people's service.' (Morrison & Wonnacott, 2009)

Although this comment relates to children's services, it is applicable across the social care field and it is this belief that underpins the content within this reader and training programme.

References

Brandon M, Dodsworth J & Rumball D (2005) Serious case reviews: learning to use expertise. *Child Abuse Review* **14** (3)160–176.

Brandon M, Belderson P, Warren C, Gardner R, Howe D, Dodsworth J & Black J (2008) The preoccupation with thresholds in cases of child death or serious injury through abuse and neglect. *Child Abuse Review* **17** (5) 313–330.

Carpenter J, Webb C, Bostock L & Coomber C (2012) *Effective Supervision in Social Work and Social Care*. London: SCIE.

McKeown K (2000) *What works in Family Support with Vulnerable Families*. Dublin: Department of Health and Children.

Morrison T (2005) *Staff Supervision in Social Care*. Brighton: Pavilion.

Morrison T & Wonnacott J (2009) Unpublished training materials.

Plymouth Safeguarding Children Board (2010) *Serious Case Review for Nursery Z*. Plymouth: Plymouth Safeguarding Children Board.

Wonnacott J (2004) *The Impact of Supervision on Child Protection Practice: A study of process and outcome*. Unpublished M.Phil University of Sussex.

Developing and Supporting Effective Staff Supervision: A reader © Pavilion Publishing and Media Ltd and its licensors 2014.

Chapter 2: An integrated approach to the delivery of supervision – the 4x4x4 model

Supervision has to address a range of requirements on behalf of different stakeholders, involving a complex set of activities. The 4x4x4 model is an integrated framework that brings together the functions, stakeholders and main processes involved in supervision. These elements have all been separately described in the literature, but the 4x4x4 model integrates them into a single model which can underpin supervision practice in a variety of settings and contexts.

The importance of the model is that it recognises the interdependence of the functions of supervision, their impact on key stakeholders and the supervision cycle as a process which ensures a focus on all the functions.

The 4x4x4 supervision model therefore brings together the:

- four key stakeholders in supervision
- four functions of supervision
- four elements of the supervisory cycle.

Table 2.1: The 4x4x4 supervision model

Four functions	Four stakeholders	Four elements of the supervision cycle
Management	People who use services	Experience
Support	Staff	Reflection
Development	The organisation	Analysis
Mediation	Partner organisations	Action planning

The four functions of supervision

The early supervision literature (Kadushin, 1976) identified three main functions of supervision: management, support and development. Later, mediation was added (Richards *et al*, 1990) as the role of the supervisor at the interface of a number of different systems became understood. These functions are integral to the definition of supervision used throughout this guide, adapted by Morrison from the work of Harries (1987), namely:

'Supervision is a process by which one worker is given responsibility by the organisation to work with another worker(s) in order to meet certain organisational, professional and personal objectives which together promote the best outcomes for service users.

The four objectives or functions of supervision are:
- *competent, accountable performance/practice (management function)*
- *continuing professional development (development function)*
- *personal support (support function)*
- *engaging the individual with the organisation (mediation function)'.*

(Morrison, 2005)

Within this definition it is important to consider the term 'management', since in some settings the main supervisory relationship is with someone other than the line manager. 'Management' is used broadly here to refer to the role that any supervisor has (whether or not they are the supervisee's line manager) in being accountable for any advice given and practice decisions that emerge from supervision. All supervisors will also have a responsibility to identify and report practice that might put a service user at risk.

Research has indicated over a number of years (eg. Gadsby Waters, 1992; Poertner & Rapp, 1983) that supervisors find it hard to pay equal attention to all four functions and that the management function may dominate. This is problematic due to the interdependency of the four functions since, for example, if it is clear that tasks are not being carried out the supervisor will need to understand why. This may involve considering whether any factors such as stress or personal issues (support), lack of confidence or skill (development) or organisational factors (mediation) are affecting performance. In other instances the support function may dominate, leading to a lack of challenge and poor performance.

The response to this tension has, in some organisations, been to separate the functions of supervision, with different supervisors being responsible for different aspects. For example, within health settings it is not unusual for a member of staff to receive clinical supervision in addition to managerial supervision and safeguarding supervision. The introduction of the restorative supervision model (Wallbank, 2013), which focuses on the emotional impact of the work and the development of worker resilience, is as a result of identifying the need to ensure that this aspect of supervision is properly addressed. Where a split approach is the preferred supervision system, attention needs to be paid to the totality of the supervisory experience of the supervisee and the risk of fragmentation and splitting between the supervisors. How will any concerns about the supervisee's practice that emerge in clinical or safeguarding supervision be addressed? How will the manager responsible for work allocation know about any personal factors or other stressors that should be taken into account? How will the roles and boundaries between the supervisors be established? **Table 2.2: Clarifying supervision arrangements across professions** sets out some of the possible permutations and issues to consider.

Table 2.2: Clarifying supervision arrangements across professions

	Single agency integrated supervision (Management/clinical/professional)	Management supervision	Clinical/professional supervision	Supervision in integrated settings
Mandate and accountability	Non-negotiable Supervisor accountable to agency	Non-negotiable Supervisor accountable to agency	Negotiated Supervisor accountable to their professional body and the agency	Negotiated by partners Supervisor accountable to partnership
Focus	Overall performance of worker	Accountability for work, time, resources, staff care, development and appraisal Communicating agency requirements	Achieving best outcomes for user Facilitating critical reflective practice	Contractual and employer oversight Plus on-site supervision of day-to-day work
Delivered by…	Single manager May be supplemented by consultation or mentoring	Manager	Professional supervisor Also via group supervision Also external approved supervisor to meet regulatory body requirements	Manager within employing agency seconding the staff member On site supervisor Professional/clinical supervision

Table 2.2: Clarifying supervision arrangements across professions (continued)

Example	Supervision of social workers within statutory social care agencies Residential and day care staff where supervision is delivered via the management structure	Supervision of staff where there are separate arrangements for clinical/professional supervision eg. OTs in multidisciplinary teams, staff in CMHTs	Provided where line management is separated from professional supervision or where the line manager is from a different profession or does not have the specific expertise required	Community mental health teams YOTs CAMHS
Issues to consider	Will all aspects of supervision receive sufficient attention? Can a focus on management tasks at the expense of reflective practice be prevented? How will the emotional impact of work and its effects on practice be addressed? How will staff be encouraged to reflect on assumptions and biases that may be influencing their work? How can specialist needs be met?	How will the organisation know about the staff's development needs? How will issues of performance feedback be addressed?	How will the supervisor be made aware of any issues that may affect practice such as workload demands? What feedback mechanism is there between the supervisor and manager? How will any differences of view between supervisor and manager be addressed?	What are the differing supervision cultures within the team? Are they understood? Where are the lines of accountability for day-to-day practice decisions? How will the emotional impact of the work be addressed across supervisory relationships?

Adapted from Morrison T (2005) *Staff Supervision in Social Care* (pp.35). Brighton: Pavilion.

One other way of thinking about how a supervisor can ensure that all four functions are addressed, while recognising that one individual supervisor cannot hope to meet all the needs of a supervisee at all the varying stages of professional development, is to think in terms of 'sharing the load'. This is different from splitting supervisor roles as there is still one supervisor, but meeting some needs is delegated to others, sometimes on a temporary basis. For example, a supervisor may ensure that a supervisee's learning and development needs are met by collaborating with others, such as trainers or mentors. They may set up shadowing arrangements and staff working in complex situations may benefit from planned consultation with particular expertise or the opportunity to engage in a series of coaching sessions. Within this approach, although significant aspects of development and support may be delegated, they will still require the supervisor's involvement since they retain overall responsibility for ensuring that the four functions of supervision are delivered.

The four stakeholders in supervision

Recognising the different functions of supervision and the interrelationship with needs of different stakeholders is essential.

The second element of the 4x4x4 model focuses on the four main stakeholders namely:

■ service users

■ supervisees

■ the organisation

■ partners, such as other organisations or professionals who also work with the same service users.

Figure 2.1: The four stakeholders identifies how the four stakeholders are interrelated and how each of their needs and activities affect those of the others. Supervision both links and influences its stakeholders.

Figure 2.1: The four stakeholders

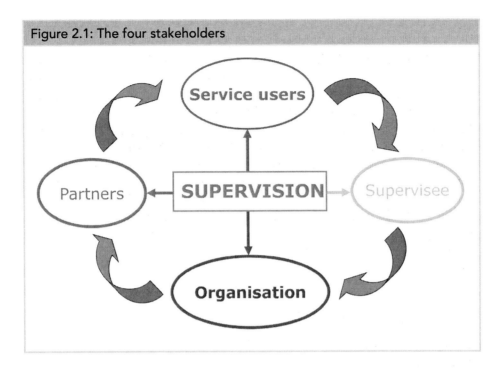

Good supervision has a positive impact on all its stakeholders, as shown in **Figures 2.2** and **2.3**.

Figure 2.2: The consequences of effective supervision

Benefits for multidisciplinary work

- Role clarity for the worker
- Identifying appropriate expectations for others
- Ensuring worker communicates with and listens to other agencies
- Preparing workers for multidisciplinary meetings
- Appreciation of different roles, challenging stereotyping
- Help workers to interpret other agencies
- Assist in mediating conflicts with other agencies, or negotiating over resources

Benefits for users

- Worker clearer, more focused
- More observant of users' strengths needs and risks
- More attentive to process and the user's feelings
- More aware of power issues
- More able to involve user
- More evidence-based assessment
- More consistent service
- Clearer plans

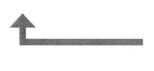

Consequences of effective supervision

Benefits for the agency

- Clearer communication both up and down
- Agency values and policies disseminated
- Increased sense of corporacy – working for the same organisation
- Improved standardisation
- Shared responsibility for problems
- Improved staff consultation processes
- Improved role understanding
- Greater openness
- Increased pride in the organisation
- Lower rates of staff turnover

Benefits for staff

- Role and accountability clear
- Work scrutinised
- Boundaries clarified
- Pressures shared
- Confidence enhanced
- Judgements reflected on
- Focus on user
- Creative practice supported
- Diversity valued
- Use/abuse of authority explored
- Poor practice challenged
- Learning needs identified
- Feelings addressed
- Worker valued, not isolated
- Team working enhanced

Figure 2.3: The consequences of poor supervision

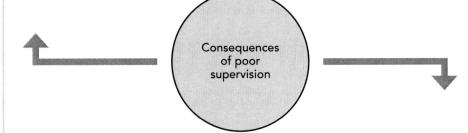

Multidisciplinary working

- Role confusion, overlap or role gap
- Information distorted or lost
- Misrepresentation of agency priorities and capacities
- Negative stereotyping of other agencies
- Simple interagency problems worsen: siege mentality

Consequences for users

- Worker less clear or prepared
- Poorer observations/listening
- Reduced empathy
- Boundaries less clear
- Assumptions unchallenged
- Inadequate assessments
- Lack of partnership
- Needs and risks not identified
- Increased turnover of workers
- Inappropriate use of authority
- Lack of user-focus

Consequences of poor supervision

Organisational communication/ cohesion

- Poor dissemination of policy
- Decreased policy compliance
- Staff unaligned with agency goals
- Mismatch of priorities
- Inter-grade relations more tense
- More conflict: grievances, etc.
- Lack of consultation with staff
- Reduced problem-solving
- Agency less user-centred
- Retention and recruitment problems
- Strategic planning weakened by lack of field level information
- Blame culture
- Loss of confidence/trust in agency

Staff

- Reduced confidence
- Unclear expectations
- Lack of accountability
- Reduced competence
- Defensive practice
- Difference perceived as threat
- Professional development impaired
- Judgements unchallenged
- Feelings unprocessed
- Isolation
- Increased sickness and staff turnover
- Dysfunctional team dynamics
- Inappropriate worker autonomy

The key here is that while there may only be two stakeholders physically present in supervision (the supervisor and supervisee) almost invariably other stakeholders are also involved and affected by what happens in supervision. Therefore, one important task for the supervisor is to ensure that other stakeholders are kept in mind and engaged within the process.

The supervision cycle

This is the third element of the 4x4x4 model and focuses on the process of supervision itself and its relationship with practice. The problem-solving supervision diagram in **Figure 2.4** is actually made up of two cycles: the 'story' or practice cycle and the supervision cycle of experience, reflection, analysis and planning.

These parallel cycles describe the process of effective practice with service users and effective supervision, and show how they are intimately related.

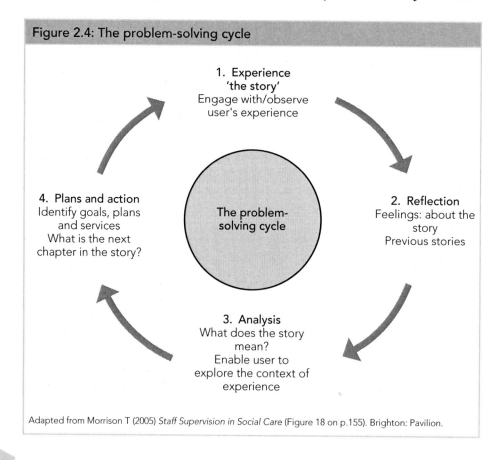

Figure 2.4: The problem-solving cycle

1. Experience
'the story'
Engage with/observe
user's experience

2. Reflection
Feelings: about the
story
Previous stories

3. Analysis
What does the story
mean?
Enable user to
explore the context of
experience

4. Plans and action
Identify goals, plans
and services
What is the next
chapter in the story?

The problem-solving cycle

Adapted from Morrison T (2005) *Staff Supervision in Social Care* (Figure 18 on p.155). Brighton: Pavilion.

The 'story' or practice cycle

This cycle shows that good practice in any setting occurs when the worker:

- engages with the service user and their story and identifies the stories of other people who are involved
- helps the user to identify the feelings generated by the story, and the feelings of others involved
- helps the user to consider the meaning of the story, its causes, consequences and impact
- helps the user to think about how they would like the next chapter of the story to be written, and what help they need to move the story on.

Experience: eliciting the story

Engaging the user at the outset is crucial in creating the context for exploring their situation. This will involve the worker in being clear about their role as well as being emotionally attentive, so that the user feels able to describe their situation and talk openly about their needs, anxieties, risks, difficulties and hopes.

Often this will involve engaging with multiple stories, such as those of different family members, and will include the worker's observation, as well as their own responses and actions. Finally, the worker will need to seek information from other organisations who are involved, thus providing an extra dimension to the story.

Reflection: the feelings about the story

Vulnerable service users may face situations and needs that are accompanied by powerful and sometimes conflicting emotions, between family members or others such as friends or neighbours. The worker needs to provide a sense of containment and security so that the emotional content of their stories can be addressed without it overwhelming the user.

However, the user's feelings and responses to the current story are often compounded by previous unresolved stories of loss or powerlessness. These earlier stories may include patterns, habits or learned responses such as the inability to trust, which have created further difficulties and complicate the current story.

It is important for the worker to help the user identify how these earlier stories or patterns may contribute to the current situation. Equally, there may also be earlier stories or experiences of resilience, courage or care that act as potential strengths or protective factors. These adaptive and pro-social patterns are just as important to explore.

Analysis: understanding the meaning of the story

It is essential for the worker to hear how the individual understands and attaches meaning to their story. What sense does the individual make of their situation, and how do they explain it, not only to the worker but also to themselves? It will include how the individual perceives the triggers, consequences and impact of their situation.

Crises often raise unspoken questions about an individual's sense of identity, self-worth, social role and future standing in their family or community. These perceptions are often bound around social and cultural expectations connected with gender, ethnicity, health, disability or class. Services and interventions cannot be planned without awareness of the social and psychological meaning of the story to those involved.

Plans and action: the next chapter of the story

This is about working with the user to identify their needs, developing tailored plans and instilling motivation and optimism for the future. Using the story metaphor, this stage involves exploring different storylines for the next chapter, re-scripting the current characters, introducing new characters, and identifying who should/could play what roles in the new story. As the next chapter unfolds and services are delivered, a further round of the cycle begins, adding new elements to the story.

In the real world, workers are usually dealing with multiple story cycles, only some of which they may know or understand. Other agencies may also be engaged, and their workers will have developed their own stories about the user.

The supervision cycle as a model for reflective supervision

The same four stages of the cycle can be applied to the supervision process. The way in which the supervisor asks questions is as important as the way the worker elicits the user's story. Open-ended questions about the user and the context will generate a very different account of what happened than closed questions with a narrow focus. In other words, the worker's account and focus are shaped significantly by the questions asked by the supervisor.

Experience of training supervisors over a number of years has shown that developing skills in asking open questions needs constant re-enforcement especially at times of stress or anxiety.

Experiencing

The origins of the supervision cycle lie in a theory of adult learning. According to Kolb (1984), learning is triggered by experience, either in terms of a problem to be solved, a situation that is unfamiliar, or a need that must be satisfied. Learning involves transforming experience into feelings (reflection), knowledge, attitudes and values (analysis), behaviours and skills (plans and action).

In professional terms, the cycle is triggered when the worker experiences a problem when undertaking a practice task, or when they identify a need such as practice development. Alternatively, the supervisor may trigger the cycle by asking the worker to review a case, or by seeking improved performance.

To make use of experience and to learn from it, there first has to be an engagement in that experience. For instance, the worker may complete the task while being psychologically disengaged with it. At this stage of the cycle, the task for the supervisor is to help the worker obtain accurate observations of what went on, and the nature of the user's circumstances. It cannot be assumed that, because the worker was present, accurate observations were made. Nor can it be assumed that in a busy office, when the supervisor asks 'What happened?' this will elicit a full account of the worker's observations. Instead, 'What happened?' may be shorthand for 'I only want to address urgent or high-risk matters, or offer immediate guidance'.

The account of practice comes as a result of the dialogue between supervisee and supervisor, and is significantly influenced by the ways in which the supervisor conducts that discussion and by the types of questions asked. Therefore, the practice cycle does not exist as an objective piece of information. Rather, the way in which the supervisor asks about the worker's observations shapes both the focus and scope of the practice account.

Reflecting

Engaging in experience is not sufficient. Without reflecting on the experience, it may be lost or misunderstood. For instance, the worker may have been engaged in a powerful piece of work but if the experience is not de-briefed or reflected on, its benefit may be lost or misunderstood.

Processing feelings often reveals a richer layer of observations, for example, observations held at an emotional level. Reflection explores feelings, patterns, and connections arising from the experience. It is also through emotion that workers identify what values or assumptions are triggered by a piece of work.

The nature of the social care task can produce strong emotional and moral responses that need to be acknowledged and processed. It is also important to clarify the source of these responses. Sometimes we feel before we see. For instance, gut reactions or feelings that can't be initially rationalised are sometimes clues to vital information about unspoken situations or dangers. When these are explored in supervision, the unconscious observations that resulted in these reactions can be uncovered.

Supervisor: 'So what was happening during the home visit at the point when you began to feel cold and shivery?'

Worker: 'Thinking back, it was when I was walking up the path and heard the dogs growling and David shouting at Annie to get his tea now.'

Such responses also need to be explored to check whether they are contaminated by the worker's personal experiences. For workers facing new demands and levels of responsibility, the opportunity to talk about the emotional demands of the work is particularly important and it is crucial that they pick up the positive message that talking about emotions is a sign of strength and competence.

Reflection allows us to recognise common elements in different situations by referencing our previous experiences. This helps workers to identify key issues quickly, along with early warning signs, priorities and tasks.

Analysis

Reflection should lead to analysis. If the cycle stops at reflection, false and subjective conclusions may be drawn. Analysis ensures that evidence and feelings are located within an external body of knowledge, theory, research and professional value, and then tested against it. For example, the reflections of a white, male practitioner about working with a black client who appears resistant, might be re-assessed when exposed to research on the wider experiences of black people in the criminal justice system.

Analysis translates information and observations into professional evidence. This occurs through interrogating information and probing discrepancies so that its meaning and significance can be elicited. It is how workers make sense of the situation and of their own assessment, intentions and plans. In doing so, analysis must incorporate the meaning of the situation to the user, as well as to the worker or their organisation. Analysis is essential in explaining and justifying intervention in people's lives, advocating resources or seeking external authority for action.

From a development perspective, analysis provides the basis for wider learning through generalisations that can be made from analysis done on a specific case. If this analysis is not done, and the worker moves straight from reflection to action, it is possible to get it 'right' without knowing why. Equally, if no analysis is done and things go wrong, it is impossible to understand why. This will prevent workers from being able to learn from difficulties or to improve their practice.

Action planning

In order to deliver effective services, the analysis needs to be translated into plans and actions. At this stage in the supervision cycle, the focus is on the planning, preparation and rehearsal of strategies.

Goals need to be set and practical options examined. Before the worker tries out a new approach or a change of tack, the supervisor may need to go through the plan with them, facilitate co-working or identify contingency plans. The supervisor's skills are important here, helping to generate and test different options. Finally, as strategies are put into action, the cycle moves into its next phase as a new experience is created and a fresh cycle begins.

Avoiding short circuits and quick fixes

The supervision process can therefore be seen as a continuous cycle of experience, reflection, analysis, planning, action and review. For problem solving or development to be fully effective, all four parts of the learning cycle need to be addressed. The challenge for supervisors is to resist the temptation and/or pressure to move rapidly from experience to plan, with little or no focus on reflection and analysis. This is the 'short circuit'. As shown in **Figure 2.5: The quick fix**, rushing or skipping the reflective and analytical stages of this process might provide a quick fix solution, but also increases the likelihood of the problem recurring as it has not been sufficiently addressed.

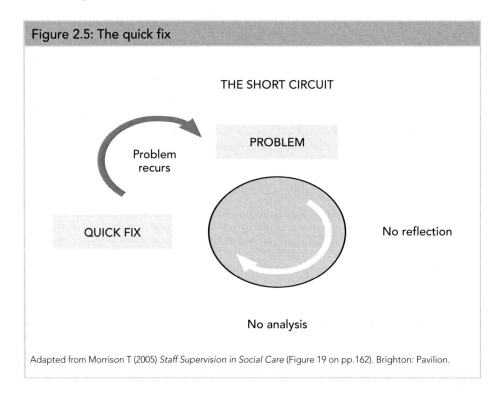

Figure 2.5: The quick fix

THE SHORT CIRCUIT

PROBLEM

Problem recurs

QUICK FIX

No reflection

No analysis

Adapted from Morrison T (2005) *Staff Supervision in Social Care* (Figure 19 on pp.162). Brighton: Pavilion.

In addition, workers have different styles and preferences, so that while one social worker may engage easily in questions about feelings, another will find this much harder. Factors such as the social worker's level of professional development, discipline, role, gender, language and class all contribute to their problem-solving style.

Using the cycle to develop reflective practice: the four levels of reflection

Reflection is a term that can be over-used and under-defined. It is a useful and practical concept only when supervisors and staff use shared language about what it is, why it is important and what evidence will show that supervisors and staff are engaged in reflection.

Reflection involves facts, feelings, assumptions, norms, values, attitudes and perceptions. Although it is an internal activity, it requires engagement with the perspectives and concerns of other stakeholders – colleagues, users, agencies or the community. Reflection makes connections between situations, contexts, roles and actions. It involves the past, present and future as well as personal, professional, political and philosophical frames of reference.

At its core, reflection is a process of creating and clarifying the meaning of experience in terms of self and self in relation to the world.

Ruch (2000) identifies four levels of reflection:

- technical
- practical
- process
- critical.

Technical reflection

Technical reflection involves the comparison of performance in practice with standards, policies or procedures and is a pragmatic form of reflection using external/technical information to identify the correct form of action. At the macro level, a performance management audit or inspection could be thought of as a formal, organisational, technical reflection.

Practical reflection

Practical reflection draws on the work of Schon (1983) who critiqued an emphasis of technical rationality and explored the role of reflection in human services where workers are often working in ill-defined and messy situations or the 'swampy lowlands'. Schon's main focus was on the individual practitioner both reflecting in action (during a practice event) and reflecting on action (reviewing experiences after the event). Thompson and Thompson (2008) add to this reflection for action ie. reflection which involved anticipating difficulties and planning ahead. This approach recognises that professional knowledge is not absolute; instead it provides a frame of reference for the practitioner that can be adapted to specific circumstances.

Process reflection

Process reflection has its roots in psychodynamic theory and the focus is on the interaction of thoughts and feelings, and how these shape the practitioner's judgements and decisions. One aim of process reflection is to increase the practitioner's awareness of the nature, source and impact of the unconscious intra- and interpersonal forces acting on them. Sheppard (2006) describes it as means to explore the assumptions, tacit knowledge and underlying theories that practitioners use. This includes raising awareness of how the practitioner's knowledge has been shaped by cultural and political forces and of the practitioner's hidden assumptions.

Critical reflection

Critical reflection takes the scrutiny of the professional's knowledge and practice one step further. It encourages practitioners to question and challenge existing power relations, and to examine how knowledge about practice is created, in whose interests and for what motives (Fook, 2002). It assumes that knowledge is formed socially rather than being neutral or objective, so it can only ever be partial and evolving. At the same time, it offers a process for challenging discussions about the experiences of practitioners and service users and the power relations between them.

The four levels of reflection are like peeling the layers of an onion, each layer deepening the level of analysis. Using these four levels leads to reflective practitioners who can provide an explanation of how they perform and a theory of action. This has the additional benefit of being able to transfer their skills and adapt existing theories and practice to a new situation.

Finally, critically reflective practitioners possess a rich mix of normative, interpretative and critical theory, which allows them to question continuously and revise their theories, as well as pay attention to the moral and ethical aspects of practice. They are also aware of the wider role that practice is fulfilling and the kind of society that their work is reproducing or changing.

It is through moving between the four stages of the supervision cycle that both supervisor and supervisee are able to engage in all four levels of reflection. However, in practice, there is often a lot of overlap between levels. A supervisory conversation may start off at one level and then move to another level. Below are examples of the four levels, showing how the supervisor may move to another level by changing the focus, perspective or purpose of the conversation. In this way, the supervisory process moves from surface to deep forms of reflection.

From technical to practical/process reflection

If the supervisor checks whether a worker has completed an assessment task within required timescales, the level is technical. The purpose is compliance monitoring, the focus is on task (completion of this assessment) and the perspective is organisational. This level of reflection is very similar to the short circuit described earlier, namely that a problem leads directly to a response. However, if the supervisor used this example to illustrate the worker's general difficulty in meeting deadlines, this would represent a move to another level of focus. This could either be on the practical level of reflection, 'What can we do about this?' or on the process level, 'Why do you think this is happening?'

From practical to process reflection

The supervisor helps a worker to think about how to structure a report. Here the level of focus is pragmatic, assisting the social worker to solve a problem and the perspective widens to include professional and user considerations. However, if the supervisor asks the worker to reflect on any anxieties about report writing and what writing reports means to them, this would be a move to the process level.

From process to critical reflection

The supervisor observes how the worker's report refers to a service user in a negative way. The supervisor asks the worker to talk about how he/she feels about the service user and how the user might find the worker and this report. Further discussion could include asking the worker to reflect on whether this user reminds them of anyone else or of a previous case. In this way, the focus of reflection moves to a personal perspective and the purpose now moves to promoting self-awareness and empathy for the service user's experience. This example would move to a critically reflective level if the supervisor asked the worker to think about how reports on service users raise wider issues about power-knowledge relations, accountability and transparency. Another example would be where a worker's reports contained assumptions, based on race, culture, class etc. for instance, about the parents of children who are unaccompanied asylum seekers. This would widen the reflective process to include a focus on how knowledge is created and how the social context influences the worker's attitudes.

Example of critical reflection

A supervisor working in a multidisciplinary service for disabled children invites the team to explore different models of disability and, in particular, the differences between medical and social models. Critical reflection has a liberating aspect to it as it provides the opportunity to challenge existing power-knowledge relations. Critical reflection explores the nature of the underlying assumptions or implicit theories of action, for example, that the abuse of disabled children is tolerated more than abuse of non-disabled children. Critical reflection asks in whose interest forms of knowledge have been created and how the construction of knowledge reproduces certain forms of social relations, for example, who wins and who loses by a particular construction of disability. Hence the perspective now widens to include public and social spheres and includes an exploration of wider social attitudes toward disability, the 'worth' of the individual and its impact on thresholds for intervention.

When workers can practise in this manner, they surely meet the definition of the reflective practitioner who, according to Sheppard (1998):

'...is aware of the socially situated relationship with their clients; has a clear understanding of their role and purpose; who understands themselves as a participant whose actions and interactions are part of the social work *process; who is capable of analysing situations and evidence, with an awareness of the way their own experience affects this process; who can identify the intellectual and practice processes involved in assessment and intervention; who is aware of the assumptions underlying the ways they make sense of practice situations; and who is able to do so in relation to the nature and purpose of their practice.'*

Although this quote relates to social worker supervision, it has a much wider application and is arguably relevant to any practitioner working within the human services.

What do we mean by reflective supervision?

It is clear from the discussion above that reflective practice is a multi-layered, essential activity if we are going to be able to work effectively with the complexity of human relationships. In recognition of this, the need for 'reflective supervision' has entered the social care language although without a consistent understanding of what this means. For example, for some it appears to be aligned to technical reflection (did I follow the correct process?); for others it is aligned to Schon's refection-on-action (stepping back and reflecting on a practice episode); for others it is focusing on emotions, whereas for others it is about reflecting on their own beliefs and attitudes and continuously questioning the basis of the knowledge they are using to inform actions.

For the purposes of this text, reflective supervision combines all of the above and is a process within which the supervisor engages with the supervisee to:

■ explore their practice and the factors that are influencing their responses (including emotional impact, power relations and social context)

■ develop a shared understanding of the knowledge base informing their analysis of any given situation and the limitations of their thinking

■ use this understanding to inform next steps.

Reflective supervision therefore engages with feelings, thoughts and actions and will automatically be promoted by effective use of the whole supervision cycle.

References

Fook J (2002) *Social Work: Critical theory and practice*. London: Sage.

Gadsby Waters J (1992) *The Supervision of Child Protection Work*. Aldershot: Avebury.

Harries (1987) cited in Morrison T (2005) *Staff Supervision in Social Care*. Brighton: Pavilion.

Kadushin A (1976) *Supervision in Social Work*. New York: Columbia University Press.

Kolb D (1984) *Experiential Learning: Experience as a source of learning and development*. London: Prentice-Hall.

Morrison T (2005) *Staff Supervision in Social Care*. Brighton: Pavilion.

Poertner J & Rapp C (1983) What is social work supervision? *The Clinical Supervisor* **1** (2) 53–65.

Richards M, Payne C & Sheppard A (1990) *Staff Supervision in Child Protection Work*. London: National Institute of Social Work.

Ruch G (2000) Self and social work: towards an integrated model of learning. *Journal of Social Work Practice* **14** (2) 99–112.

Schon D (1983) *The Reflective Practitioner: How professionals think in action*. Aldershot: Arena.

Sheppard M (1998) Practice validity reflexivity and knowledge for social work. *British Journal of Social Work* **28** 763–781.

Sheppard M (2006) *Social Exclusion and Social Work: The idea of practice*. Aldershot UK: Ashgate.

Thompson S & Thompson N (2008) *The Critically Reflective Practitioner*. Palgrave MacMillan: Basingstoke.

Wallbank S (2013) Recognising stressors and using restorative supervision to support a healthier maternity workforce: a retrospective, cross-sectional, questionnaire survey. *Evidence Based Midwifery* **11** (1) 4–9.

Chapter 3: Developing the supervisory relationship

Carpenter *et al*'s (2012) review of the supervision research identified a number of components that underpin the best supervision. These were:

- social and emotional support
- a supervisor with expert knowledge
- task assistance
- reflective space
- a positive relationship.

The importance of an effective relationship is a theme throughout this reader and although most supervisors and supervisees would not argue with this, it may feel hard to achieve. Research and surveys consistently show that supervisees frequently experience supervision as focused on task completion rather than providing a relationship where support, reflection and their own development is a priority. For example, a Community Care Survey in June 2013 reported that:

- 37.5% of respondents said they did not receive supervision because 'it is not prioritised in my organisation'
- 54% of respondents said none of their supervision was reflective – while 28% said the reflective elements made up roughly half
- 73% of respondents said supervision was about monitoring targets and timescales.

Supervisors may feel pulled between a desire to spend time and energy developing a collaborative relationship which provides the safety and containment required for the worker to explore difficulties, anxieties and uncertainties on one hand, and meeting the needs of the organisation for management information and procedural compliance on the other. The development of the relationship itself may become part of the compliance with procedures, with supervision agreements becoming tick box exercises devoid of any real meaning for the individual concerned.

The effective implementation of the 4x4x4 model of supervision must be underpinned by a focus on the quality of the supervisory relationship, otherwise engagement across all elements of the supervision cycle and the balanced implementation of the functions is unlikely to be achieved. Without a safe place where they feel contained and able to reflect honestly on their practice, the worker's capacity for honesty and openness about their practice is likely to be minimised with the result that the supervisor becomes wary or suspicious about their work, leading to further defensiveness. The compromised supervision cycle described in Chapter 1 is likely to come into play, with the attendant negative impact on service user outcomes.

The components of an effective supervisory relationship identified by a recent practice enquiry undertaken by the Social Care Institute for Excellence (Lambley & Marrable, 2013) were openness, honesty and respect, including respecting the feelings of the worker. The accompanying practice guide (SCIE, 2013) goes on to note:

'In addition, the development of an effective relationship will depend upon how far the supervisor is perceived by the supervisee to meet their needs and it is important that there is a clear understanding by both parties of their role, responsibilities and the boundaries and limitations of their relationship. This understanding can be enhanced by the effective use of the supervision agreement or contract.'

One reason often cited for a failure to pay attention to the less tangible aspects of supervision, such as relationship development, is a lack of time. In fact, research and practice evidence would suggest that time paid to relationship development, particularly at the start, will pay dividends later on. Too often supervisors and supervisees can become embroiled in negative interactions and mistrust of each other when at the heart of the tension is a complex interaction of many factors, some of which are either historical or below the surface. For example, in a residential setting the new supervisee who is aware that many of the staff (including their supervisor) are from the local community and are friends outside work may also have recently come from a job where they had felt bullied by their manager. They may not open up in supervision and are therefore seen by the supervisor as negative, aloof and defensive. When the supervisee makes a minor mistake this is not shared with their supervisor who, when they find out later, sees this as confirming their concerns about the worker. This negative spiral could have been avoided by time spent understanding each other's perspective right from the start.

At the heart of such tensions may be a misunderstanding about the need to take a balanced approach in the way that authority is used and perceived within the relationship.

Authority and the supervisory relationship

Understanding role and responsibilities will include developing a common appreciation of the authority inherent in the role of supervisor. Hughes and Pengelly (1997) refer to authority within supervision as having three aspects and the best supervisors as achieving a balance across all three.

1. Role authority

This refers to the authority vested in the supervisor by the organisation. Both supervisor and supervisee need to understand and respect the boundaries of the role; for example, that part of the supervisory task is to challenge the supervisee's thinking and encourage critical reflection.

2. Personal authority

This is the authority the supervisor has by virtue of who they are and how they are perceived as a person by the supervisee. Are they someone with integrity, who can be trusted to be fair, open and honest in their dealings with others? Do they have the respect of the team and colleagues?

3. Professional authority

Supervisors will also need to have authority by virtue of their professional knowledge and expertise or their open recognition of the limits and boundaries of their knowledge and skill base. For some supervisors who may be from a different professional background to their supervisees, this last point is crucial.

Achieving a balance across these three aspects involves both supervisor and supervisee having an opportunity to get to know each other, explore their strengths and limitations and establish a professional working alliance. Two tools that can help this process and are core to the model of supervision being described within this reader are the supervision agreement/contract and the supervision history. Both are simple, effective ways of developing the relationship, and experience of working with many supervisors suggests that they can be particularly useful as a means of preventing relationship problems and turning existing problems around.

The supervision agreement

This is also sometimes referred to as the supervision contract.

Although supervision agreements have been discussed in the literature for many years (eg. Morrison, 1993), there is continuing evidence that their implementation is patchy. For example, a survey of a multi-professional group (Bell, 2009) found that almost half the respondents (49%) said that they did not have a supervision contract or agreement; with only 44% saying they did have such a contract. Staff from nursing were the most likely to have a contract (62%) and medical staff were least likely (6%). Only 37% of social work respondents had a contract.

One problem is that the agreement can be seen as yet another bureaucratic process and a form filling exercise, rather than an important step in relationship development. In fact the process of developing the agreement is as important as the final document and it should be seen as a live tool for on-going reflection on the quality and process of supervision.

Supervision agreements are important because:
■ they reflect the seriousness of the activity of supervision

■ the development of the agreement positively models partnership behaviour

- they clarify roles and responsibilities

- they clarify accountability and authority

- they are a basis for reviewing the relationship

- they are a benchmark for auditing the quality of supervision.

Supervision agreements and anti-oppressive practice

Inherent within the above is the establishment of a relationship where power, authority and the way this is exercised within supervision is made explicit and open to review. Supervision needs to be acknowledged as an authority relationship but one where there is no misuse of power. The relationship between power and authority is a complex one and complexity is increased where there are differences in gender, ethnicity, culture, language, class, sexuality or disability. In these circumstances the misuse of power can result in marginalisation or discrimination and contribute to poor practice. Fears about this affect both parties and may result in:

- supervisors who relinquish their authority because they fear it will be seen as discriminatory

- supervisees who are unwilling to respect their supervisor's legitimate authority

- supervisors who abuse their authority through not accepting differences, which may result in over-management and over-representation of staff from minority groups in grievance and disciplinary procedures

- supervisors who ignore differences and appear to treat everyone the same, which leads to others being expected to adapt to the belief system of the dominant group

- supervisors who avoid supervision on the grounds that the supervisee needs someone special, leading to the worker losing the support and guidance they are entitled to, affecting their ability to achieve and increasing marginalisation.

The process of developing a supervision agreement provides a forum within which differences can be openly acknowledged and potential issues explored. Reviewing the agreement provides an important opportunity for the supervisor to understand how their supervisee experiences their authority as well as gauge whether their supervisee feels that supervision is a place where they are challenged to look at values, power issues and partnership practice. The agreement therefore underpins anti-oppressive practice both within the supervisory relationship and in work with service users.

Negotiating an effective supervision agreement

One way of thinking about the agreement is as a three-legged stool with three elements that all need to be in place for the stool to remain sturdy and upright.

These three elements are:

- administrative – frequency, location, recording
- professional – purposes, focus, principles, accountabilities
- psychological – motivation, trust, commitment, ownership, investment.

A five-stage framework for negotiating the agreement

Moving beyond the agreement as a quick form filling exercise, this approach focuses on the overall process with the written document being the end product rather than the process itself. The five stages are:

1. mandate
2. engagement
3. acknowledging ambivalence
4. written agreement
5. reviewing the agreement

Mandate

Both supervisor and supervisee need to know from the outset what the mandate for supervision is and clarify the nature of the authority vested in the supervisor by the organisation.

Key issues to discuss at the mandate stage:

- What does the employer's policy state about the expectations of supervision?
- How does this policy relate to standards set by professional bodies?
- What is non-negotiable?
- What is negotiable?
- What rights are there for each person in supervision?
- What responsibilities does each person have in supervision?
- What are the boundaries and limits to confidentiality?
- What records are to be maintained, who keeps them, who can see them and for what purposes?

Engagement

A clear mandate for supervision is the foundation, but it does not necessarily guarantee engagement by either party. There still needs to be a psychological mandate, providing a shared perception and commitment to supervision by both people, based on agreed roles, responsibilities, needs and expectations. With this engagement, both parties can start to build trust, reduce anxiety and increase certainty about supervision.

Engagement does not occur overnight. It requires time, mutual trust and understanding. The process of getting to know each other can be greatly helped by focusing on specific engagement issues. This helps to clarify where each person is coming from professionally and what influences their approach both to practice and supervision. Addressing these areas up front can help build a fruitful and collaborative supervision relationship.

Areas to explore at the engagement stage include:

- previous training and supervisory experiences, and their effects on the way each perceives and approaches supervision
- what the worker would find helpful from the supervisor in the light of their previous experiences of supervision and the expectations of the social worker's programme
- how might the supervisor notice that the supervisee is anxious or stressed?

- expectations around the handling of authority and conflict within supervision

- the learning styles of the supervisee and the degree to which this matches the learning style of the supervisor

- the beliefs and values each bring about the nature, purpose and rationale of the work

- any factors relating to gender, class, race, culture, sexual orientation, disability etc. that might impact on the supervisory relationship

- each party's approach to user participation and the use of authority in practice.

This list includes areas for both supervisor and supervisee to explore. Building the relationship is not simply about the supervisor understanding the supervisee, but also the supervisee understanding the supervisor. For instance, if the supervisee brings a strongly risk averse approach to their practice but the supervisor is strongly risk tolerant, this needs to be acknowledged and discussed early on.

Acknowledging ambivalence

Workers in the helping professions will inevitably experience strong emotions related to:

- personal impact of the work causing sadness, despair, confusion or fear

- over-identification with certain users or situations

- intolerance or moral disgust at the user's situation or behaviour

- frustration or demoralisation at the lack of time or resources available

- mismatch of positive expectations about the job with its realities.

In addition to these, Claxton (1988) states that adults are ambivalent about learning and development because they carry irrational beliefs about themselves. These beliefs are particularly strong in the helping professions and workers may feel a pressure to prove their skills and worth to their new employer and colleagues. They may feel:

- I must be competent

- I must be in control

- I must be consistent

- I must be comfortable.

Each new supervisory relationship is an unknown quantity, and both parties have to take some level of risk. This is especially true for the worker, who may encounter areas where they feel both less competent and comfortable, and where they fail to act consistently. These may have been unrecognised aspects of the supervisee's experience or located at a level below their conscious awareness. Exploring these emotions and ambiguities in supervision offers some of the best developmental opportunities. It is also possible that the worker's discomfort may reflect wider processes at play within the team, organisation or with other agencies.

There are real benefits to exploring issues around emotion and ambivalence and this can lead to a much deeper level of analysis. However, the supervisee may be very apprehensive about exploring such issues, fearing that they will be perceived as unable to cope, or even incompetent. It is therefore very important that the supervisor normalises these responses and may, for example, say:

'I know this work generates strong emotional and attitudinal responses. The triggers vary with each of us, as does the way that we deal with such situations and especially how they surface in supervision. In order for me to know how to respond most helpfully, could you say something about what happens when you feel out of your depth, confused, distressed, scared or angry? What would I notice as a supervisor that would alert me to this? What would you find helpful in such situations?"

However, the reality is that such an exploration can lead to tensions in the relationship. Acknowledging this likelihood at the start establishes the fact that supervision may feel uncomfortable or challenging at times and that this is to be expected. It is important as part of this discussion to explore the avenues open to either party if they feel the relationship is becoming stuck and tensions are preventing supervision from supporting high quality practice.

Written agreement

A structured approach to forming a supervisory agreement will motivate both parties to be proactive and considered in making their expectations a reality. However, these discussions need to be translated into specific written agreements. Whatever format is used, it will need to:

- be arrived at through negotiation
- address issues and how they will be managed
- be co-signed and dated

- be copied for both supervisor and supervisee
- be reviewed at least annually.

Reviewing the agreement

Too often a supervision agreement will be put in a drawer and forgotten. The review process is, however, vital as relationships do not remain static and will change over time in response to both internal and external factors. Reviewing the agreement provides an opportunity to consider the health of the supervisory relationship from the perspective of both parties, prevent inertia and keep a focus on the importance of supervision.

The supervision history

The supervision history is a fundamental aspect of relationship development and feeds into the engagement stage of the agreement process. This tool acknowledges that the supervisee's responses to supervision will be affected by their previous experiences and provides a framework for the supervisor and supervisee to understand these. The supervisor's own responses and style as a supervisor will be similarly affected by their own history and the most successful supervision cultures are established where all staff throughout the organisation have had the opportunity to reflect on their own histories of being supervised and understand how these affect them in both their supervisor and supervisee roles.

This process should, however, be optional; workers should have the opportunity to opt out and be able to reflect on the questions in private first. In close-knit organisations there may be a reluctance to talk about past supervisors who may be easily identifiable and time will need to be given to establishing the confidential nature of the discussion, as well as agreeing how to refer to the individual involved (eg. using numbers or initials).

Taking a history

Supervisees are invited to:

- write out a list of previous supervisors, including significant figures such as previous managers, mentors or teachers
- make a brief note about their impact; did they help in professional development? If so, in what ways?

- identify what it was about their style, focus, practice, understanding, knowledge, skills, values, use of authority, empathy or any other factors that influenced them

- consider how the style of supervision had an impact on practice and relationships with colleagues.

The answers to these questions are discussed and the supervisor and supervisee explore what needs to happen to ensure their supervision relationship is supportive, focused and purposeful.

The benefits of this tool are:

- it provides a forum to explore in a non-threatening way power issues and the use of authority

- it allows for the identification of any vulnerabilities as well as coping styles

- it allows the supervisor to understand any significant professional influences

- it establishes that making the relationship work is a shared responsibility

- it allows the supervisor to identify and understand any blocks to learning and development.

Working with transition

Developing the supervisory relationship will include understanding the many factors that might be affecting the supervisee and one such crucial factor is change and transition. Since continual change is a constant feature of work within the human services, a model is used here to assist supervisors in understanding and working with situations where their supervisees may be new to a role or experiencing changes to their working environment. An understanding of transition may help in deepening the discussion at the stage of developing an agreement, taking a supervision history or working with the relationship through a time of change.

It could be argued that unless the supervisor has paid proper attention to all the factors that might be affecting the relationship they are unlikely to understand the full impact that transition will have on their supervisee.

Figure 3.1: Transition in the workplace explores the possible impact of taking on a new role. At each stage there will be challenges for the supervisee. Their capacity to articulate their feelings and ask for appropriate help will be affected by a range of factors which may be socio-cultural (eg. men do not ask for help), organisational/professional (eg. help-seeking is a sign of weakness) or personal (eg. last time I asked for help I was seen as incompetent). The challenge for the supervisor is to understand the implications of this process.

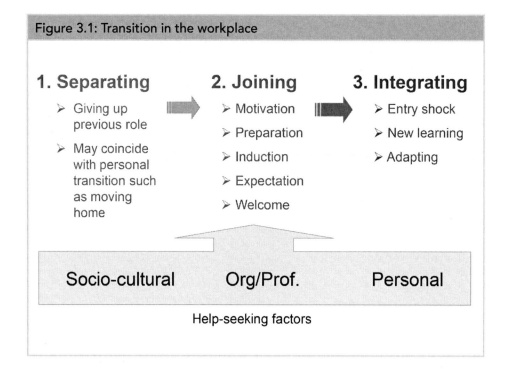

Figure 3.1: Transition in the workplace

1. Separating
➢ Giving up previous role
➢ May coincide with personal transition such as moving home

2. Joining
➢ Motivation
➢ Preparation
➢ Induction
➢ Expectation
➢ Welcome

3. Integrating
➢ Entry shock
➢ New learning
➢ Adapting

Socio-cultural   Org/Prof.   Personal

Help-seeking factors

The transition curve

This model (Nye, 2007) can be used to describe a wide variety of changes at both group and individual levels. In essence, the model suggests that initial excitement at taking up a new job or role quickly gives way to shock, anxiety and even immobilisation at the reality of workplace demands.

Figure 3.2: Period of transition

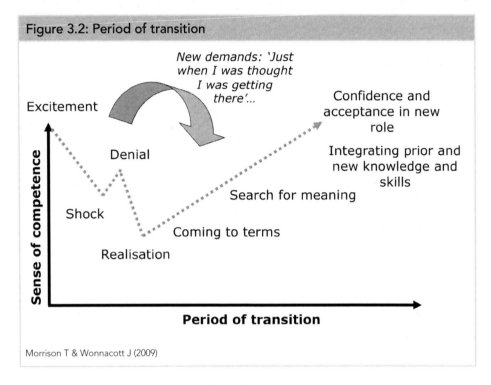

Morrison T & Wonnacott J (2009)

In response, the worker's sense of confidence and competence drop. In some cases, a defence against this might be denial, in which the worker presents themselves as confident, even over-confident, to ward off the underlying anxiety. With solid support, the worker can begin to accept and come to terms with the new reality. This allows them to engage more fully with the experience, and start to work out what working in the new role actually means.

Through gradual exposure to a wider range of tasks and responsibilities, combined with learning and development opportunities, the integration of previous knowledge and workplace know-how deepens. Together, these processes help the worker to develop their professional confidence.

Figure 3.3: Negotiating identity changes shows how the performance of roles and tasks is anchored in these issues. Part of the entry shock is discovering the gap between expectations and the reality. How the worker negotiates their changing identity is therefore important in adapting to their new role and tasks.

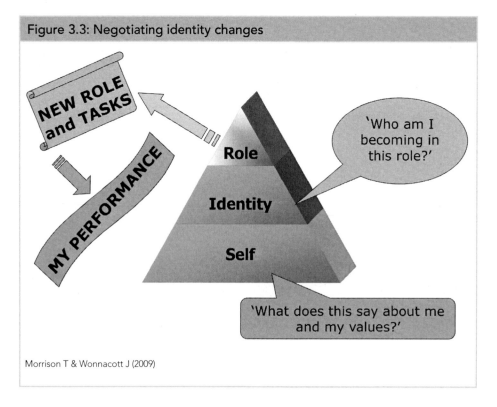

Figure 3.3: Negotiating identity changes

Morrison T & Wonnacott J (2009)

Figure 3.4 shows the shock that can accompany the early stage of transition and highlights that a successful transition to a new identity has to be negotiated. It cannot be imposed. Success in making this transition is critically dependent on the support available and supervision is a key part of this process.

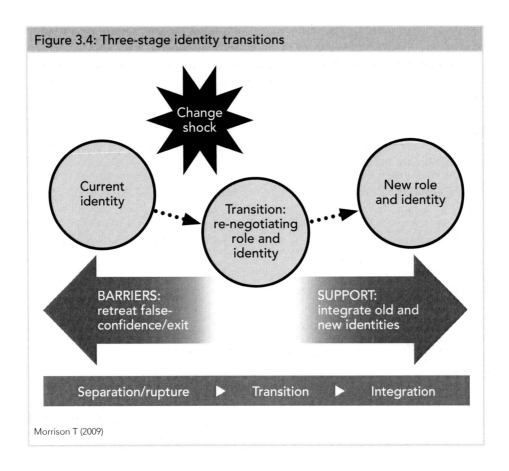

Figure 3.4: Three-stage identity transitions

Morrison T (2009)

In summary

Paying attention to the quality of the relationship between supervisor and supervisee is a fundamental aspect of the supervisory process. An effective supervisory relationship that encourages the development of the supervisee will be enhanced by the use of the supervision history and supervision agreement, both of which facilitate an understanding of each party's contribution. A vital facet of the supervisory relationship is an ability to acknowledge and understand the impact of emotion upon the supervisor, supervisee and service user, and this will be examined in Chapter 4.

References

Bell (2009) *Child Welfare Professionals' Experience of Supervision: A study of the supervision experiences of professionals who attended 2009 Congress*. York: Baspcan.

Carpenter J, Webb C, Bostock L & Coomber C (2012) *Effective Supervision in Social Work and Social Care*. London: SCIE.

Claxton (1988) *Live and Learn: An introduction to the psychology of growth and change in everyday life*. Open University Press: Milton Keynes

Community Care (2013) Third of UK's social workers not currently receiving supervision [online]. Available at: http://www.communitycare.co.uk/2013/06/18/third-of-uks-social-workers-not-currently-receiving-supervision/ (accessed October 2013).

Hughes L & Pengelly P (1997) *Staff Supervision in a Turbulent World*. London: Jessica Kingsley.

Lambley S & Marrable T (2013) *Practice Enquiry into Supervision in a Variety of Adult Care Settings where there are Health and Social Care Practitioners Working Together*. London: SCIE.

Morrison T (1993) *Staff Supervision in Social Care*. Harlow: Longman.

Morrison T & Wonnacott J (2009) Unpublished training materials.

Nye C (2007) Dependence and independence in clinical supervision: an application of Vygotsky's developmental learning theory. *The Clinical Supervisor* **26** (1/2) pp81–98.

SCIE (2013) *Effective Supervision in a Variety of Settings*. London: SCIE.

Chapter 4: Working positively with emotions in supervision

The 'support' or 'restorative' function of supervision acknowledges the importance of staff care, and the role of the supervisor in recognising and managing stress, ensuring the well-being of the worker and working with them towards the development of emotional resilience. Evidence suggests (Lambley & Marrable, 2013; Bourn & Hafford-Letchfield, 2011; Gibbs, 2001) that appropriate emotional support can be an important buffer against stress, anxiety and high workloads. In addition, exploring the meaning of emotional reactions to the work can also be an important element in managing casework, particularly in relation to risk. For example, research into working with violence and aggression found that workers who felt anxious or scared visiting families where there was a risk of violence needed the opportunity to recognise what these feelings might be saying about risks to children living within that environment (Stanley & Goddard, 2002).

One important aspect of the 4x4x4 model of supervision is that working with emotions is an integral part of the supervisory process. The restorative function of supervision is not separate but instead is seen as crucial to facilitating an approach to practice which recognises the impact that feelings have on thoughts and actions. Recognising worker stress and anxiety, as well as providing a safe environment where the emotional impact of the work can be explored, is therefore a fundamental task of the supervisor. This approach recognises emotions as a form of communication and the competence of both supervisors and supervisee in working positively with emotions will affect the quality of the supervisory process.

How emotional intelligence/ competence contributes to effective practice

Exactly what contribution does emotional competence make to effective supervision and effective practice? Also termed 'emotional intelligence', it is a way of using thinking about feelings to guide our decision-making. Mayer and Salovey (1997) in revising early definitions refer to emotional intelligence as involving:

'The ability to perceive accurately, appraise and express emotion; the ability to access and/or generate feelings when they facilitate thought; the ability to understand emotion and emotional knowledge; and the ability to regulate emotions to promote emotional and intellectual growth.' (p10)

According to Goleman *et al* (2002), it has four interrelated elements:

■ emotional awareness about one's own feelings and the sources of these feelings

■ empathy – the ability to understand what another person is or might be feeling

■ self-management – the ability to manage one's emotions to achieve one's goals

■ interpersonal skills – the ability to relate to others in a purposeful and thoughtful manner.

Another aspect of emotional competence is the 'value base', which Morrison (2007) added as an underpinning element since values shape the purpose and outcomes of how emotional competence is used. To take an extreme example, a sophisticated psychopath might have the emotional skills to manipulate our emotions, but lacks the value base which prevents this skill being used to deceive or hurt us.

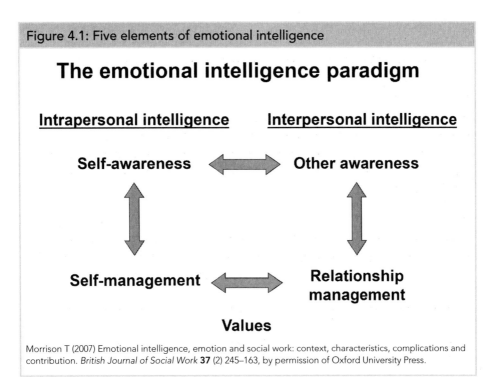

Figure 4.1: Five elements of emotional intelligence

The emotional intelligence paradigm

Intrapersonal intelligence

Interpersonal intelligence

Self-awareness ⟷ **Other awareness**

Self-management ⟷ **Relationship management**

Values

Morrison T (2007) Emotional intelligence, emotion and social work: context, characteristics, complications and contribution. *British Journal of Social Work* **37** (2) 245–163, by permission of Oxford University Press.

The arrows in **Figure 4.1** indicate how the five elements interrelate, in particular the links between self-awareness and other awareness as a basis for managing self and relationships.

Writing about the role of emotional intelligence in social work practice, Howe (2008) notes the need for social workers to reflect on how they are emotionally affected by their clients and also how they emotionally affect others. A positive supervisory relationship provides the containment and safe place where this can happen. The quality of the relationship with the supervisor is therefore crucial, as according to Howe (2008):

'Good reflective supervision can help deepen the worker's understanding of their own and their service user's psychological condition and mental state so that the therapeutic nature of the relationship between worker and user is maintained.' (p.187)

Morrison (2007) explores further the relationship between emotional intelligence, the quality of relationships with service users and the impact of these relationships on the effectiveness of services across a number of core tasks.

Engagement of service users

Work cannot be effective unless attention has first been paid to a process of engagement and rapport building with the service user.

Observation

Research shows that recall about emotional events is reduced when we try to suppress emotion (Richards & Gross, 2000). Suppressing this information can come from role confusion, personal discomfort or organisational cultures that devalue the role of emotions.

Attachment theory suggests that discomforting emotions provide signals of possible danger which require attention and appraisal. A lack of self-awareness or suppression of emotion may result in observations being missed, either about the presence of external dangers or about the impact of the social worker's unresolved personal experiences, which may compromise the assessment process. The ability to identify our own and others' emotions accurately also helps us to spot false emotions in others (Ekman, 1985).

Assessment

There is a clear link between the relationship skill of the worker and the quality of assessment. This is particularly true in relation to any matters that are morally or emotionally charged, such as trauma, loss or problematic behaviours, for example, excessive drinking or offending. Service users become quickly aware of a worker who is not in tune with their emotions. Therefore, the ability of the worker to build the necessary emotional rapport and trust, allowing for a collaborative assessment, is critical to the quality of assessment.

Decision-making

Emotions also play a significant role in decision-making (Damasio, 2006 cited in Munro, 2008):

'Emotion is integral to the processes of reasoning and decision making ... Well targeted and well deployed emotion seems to be a support system without which the edifice of reason cannot operate properly.'

In other words, rather than seeing emotions as being against reason, emotions are positioned here as being part of the whole reasoning process. There is, however, a big difference between being aware of feelings and what they are telling us, and states of high emotion that can't be explored and reflected upon.

Isen (2000) found that positive emotion is associated with a range of mental capacities that have a direct impact on judgement and decision-making, such as:

■ creative thinking

■ the ability to link between different sources and types of information

■ increased elaboration of information

■ greater flexibility in negotiation situations

■ improved diagnostic/assessment ability.

Howe (2008) argues that emotional awareness helps us to deal with uncertainty and new situations by rapidly processing information. Emotions also help us predict the future by imagining potential consequences either for ourselves or others, such as the likely impact of our interventions on service users.

Because emotion is a bridge between the known and the unknown, emotional competence plays a central role in decision making. Thinking without emotional knowledge is as problematic as emotion without thought.

Working with others

Work in the human services is a collaborative practice. It is not enough for workers to be able to work individually with their service user, or within their own setting, if they are unable to maintain healthy relationships with colleagues and partner agencies.

Workers operating in statutory settings will act as key workers responsible for co-ordinating multidisciplinary assessment and planning processes. However, the environment in which workers have to form and sustain these relationships is complex and demanding. Unhealthy organisational cultures can affect how feelings in the workplace are expressed and managed, and in these types of environment emotional competence is vital.

Isen (2000) found that positive emotion reduces inter-group hostility and discrimination, enables people to identify commonalities and makes it more likely that members will treat other groups as members of their own. Wells (2004) identifies a positive association between emotional intelligence and openness to differences. The work of both these researchers indicates that emotional competence has implications for practitioners' ability to practise and work with other agencies in an anti-discriminatory manner. Values and knowledge about discrimination must be integrated with interpersonal skills if practitioners are to be able not only to identify but also to challenge these factors appropriately.

Emotions and authoritative practice

Wonnacott (2012), building on training materials developed with Tony Morrison and In-Trac associates, explores four styles of supervision based on four styles of parenting identified by research (Baumrind, 1978; Lexmond & Reeves, 2009). Which style is employed will depend largely on the way in which the supervisor can balance their role in working positively with emotions (being responsive) with a clear focus on practice standards (being demanding).

The *authoritative* supervisor (high demand/high responsiveness) will have a high degree of emotional intelligence, feel comfortable working with emotional impact, be responsive to the worker's psychological needs and at the same time remain focused on the quality of practice that each service user should expect, and demand high standards of practice. The likely outcome is a confident, secure worker who will form effective relationships with service users and other agencies and provide high quality services.

In contrast...

The *authoritarian* supervisor (high demand/low responsiveness) will demand high standards of practice but lack emotional intelligence, and will suppress or ignore any reference to emotions, stress or anxiety. One likely outcome is a worker who becomes dependent on the supervisor and is scared to use their own professional judgement. They may become risk averse and possibly punitive or rigid in their approach to service users.

The *permissive* supervisor (low demand/high responsiveness) will be responsive to the emotional impact of the work and the supervisee's need for support but in doing so will avoid making demands and lose a focus on the needs of the service user. The outcome of this style may be a worker who lacks focus on the requirements of their role and the needs of the service user. They may become overly autonomous and possibly over-dependent on the supervisor to solve problems for them.

The *neglectful* supervisor (low demand/low responsiveness) is likely to be so bound up in their own problems and issues that they are unable to either support their supervisee effectively or be clear about expected practice standards. This situation may also occur when the supervisor overestimates the capability of the supervisee and does not prioritise their need for supervision. The supervisee in this situation is likely to become anxious, isolated and unclear about their role and without strong team support may become burnt out. Their anxiety is likely to inhibit the development of effective relationships with service users and other professionals. Their practice skills may stagnate and their quality of work with service users deteriorate.

Creating a secure environment for supervision

The supervisory process sits within a wider context of team, organisational and inter-agency dynamics and will be influenced by the structures and cultures of these wider networks. In order to support staff, especially new workers, and to provide a safe, predictable and focused supervisory process, it is important to be aware of how wider organisational and inter-agency forces can impact on supervision. This section provides a model for understanding this by looking at the impact of anxiety, change and uncertainty on organisational behaviour.

The impact of organisational anxiety and uncertainty on supervision

Anxiety and uncertainty are common realities in human services, given the complex and often uncertain nature of the work, the continuous change and the extensive scrutiny. This cannot be eliminated through procedures or training, and there is a need to think about how organisations, not just individuals, address anxiety and uncertainty. Managing anxiety and uncertainty is a crucial task. **Figure 4.2: The impact of organisational**

anxiety on supervision shows two very different ways in which organisations can respond to anxiety. In the red (outer) cycle there is the compromised environment and in the green (middle) cycle there is the collaborative environment. In the yellow (central) cycle, we see the supervision cycle described in Chapter 2.

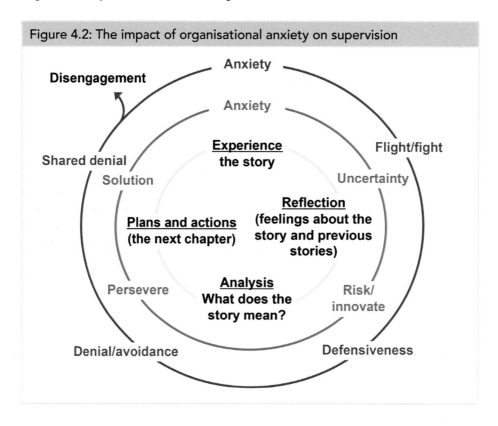

Figure 4.2: The impact of organisational anxiety on supervision

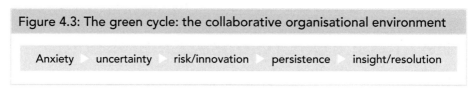

Figure 4.3: The green cycle: the collaborative organisational environment

Anxiety ▸ uncertainty ▸ risk/innovation ▸ persistence ▸ insight/resolution

The green cycle can also be thought of as the collaborative organisational environment, which is most likely to support effective supervision.

The collaborative organisational environment provides this through:

- clear organisational values and goals
- positive and engaged leadership
- clear policies, procedures and standards
- a robust performance management framework
- effective workforce development and training
- open communication within the organisation
- active participation with and from service users
- positive structures for inter-agency work.

In the green cycle, the uncertainties and anxieties associated with continuous change and the nature of the work are openly acknowledged. This is a culture that values the expression of healthy uncertainty, feelings and difference. It is an environment where problems and mistakes are grasped as opportunities for learning rather than punishment. The culture recognises that there are rarely simple or prescribed solutions for managing complexity and risk, and creativity and innovation are valued. It is possible for workers to take a risk and express doubts, reveal difficulties and share practice, as well as try out new approaches.

Power relations are made explicit, diversity is valued, and roles and responsibilities are clarified. Difficult problems are openly acknowledged and there is a shared commitment to grapple and persist with these issues.

People are also not expected or allowed to go it alone. In such a climate, staff are able to learn from their experience, deepening their practice and developing creative and sometimes unexpected solutions. As a result, confidence and skills to tackle new challenges are increased.

Features of the green team environment

- Respectful attitude and concern for service users.
- Roles and responsibilities are clear.

- Staff show sense of belonging, mutual support and shared responsibility.

- Clear and open communication.

- Positive engagement with external agencies.

- Commitment to resolve conflicts, including those with other agencies.

- Feelings acknowledged and used to explore practice.

- Difference acknowledged and valued.

- Supervision seen as a priority.

- Theory and research used to assist practice.

- Staff committed to learning and development.

- Positive use of team meetings.

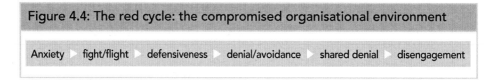

Figure 4.4: The red cycle: the compromised organisational environment

Anxiety ▶ fight/flight ▶ defensiveness ▶ denial/avoidance ▶ shared denial ▶ disengagement

In sharp contrast, the red cycle depicts an environment in which anxiety is seen as a sign of weakness and a threat to the organisation that can't be acknowledged. In this culture, workers are expected to be professionals and to cope, regardless of the pressure of work or organisational change. As a result, problems and uncertainties are suppressed. Initially this is through fight or flight mechanisms, such as conflict, grievances, sickness and high staff turnover. There is a transfer of internal conflict onto external relationships with other agencies.

The lack of spaces within the organisation where uncertainty and difference can be explored leads to defensiveness and avoidance. Working parties fail to complete their tasks and issues remain unaddressed. There is a fear of exposing practice, often based on real experience, because the only time practice is audited is when something has gone wrong and there is a search for a scapegoat. In such environments, it is neither safe to expose practice nor to declare problems, doubts or uncertainties.

Social defence systems

Workers in this environment tend to defend themselves and ward off painful realities by denying uncomfortable information and opinions. Difference is perceived as a threat and is rejected in favour of the dominant group's frame of reference. This becomes institutionalised through 'social defence systems', in which denial becomes part of workplace relations and processes, leading to a form of organisational or shared denial (Menzies-Lyth, 1970).

Characteristics of this include:

- depersonalisation

- detachment and denial of feelings

- rigid and narrow definition of task – 'just following procedures'

- constant counter-checking and lack of trust

- re-distributing responsibility through projection and blaming

- re-framing and minimising the true nature of concerns

- clinging to the familiar, even when it has stopped being functional.

If this is left unchallenged, these processes may eventually result in disengagement, with the organisation preoccupied solely with its own survival. As described by Hughes and Pengelly (1997), the needs of the service user become lost and external partners experience the organisation as a fortress with its drawbridge up. The result is real tension between what the organisation says it is doing, what the staff think they are doing and what staff are actually doing.

Features of a red cycle environment

- Absence of trust both between individuals and towards the organisation.

- Lack of leadership, strategy or planning.

- Poor communication within the organisation.

- Lack of clear policies, standards and systems.

- Low involvement and participation by the service user.

- High levels of defensiveness, blame and finding scapegoats.

- Absence of supervision or frequent cancellations.

- High level of staff turnover and/or sickness.

- Feelings acted out or denied.

- Staff becoming more and more dependent on their managers.

- Inappropriate or discriminatory humour.

- High number of staff safety incidents and staff working in unsafe settings.

- Users seen as demanding and threatening.

- Unpredictable service responses.

Consequences for supervision of the red cycle environment

In such an environment it will become less safe for supervisors or supervisees to reflect and analyse and they will strive to find security and predictability in procedures and systems. The focus will be restricted to the problem in hand and going straight for the quick fix to avoid looking below the surface at what is really going on. Supervision may become something to avoid, or to get involved with only on a bureaucratic level.

Such environments are especially damaging for new staff and may leave them cautious about engaging with supervision in the future and generally distrustful of organisational authority. Oppressive processes also go unchallenged and power structures become personalised.

When organisations stop operating in a mindful way there are consequences for staff and service users. While workers will try hard to make sure that their work is unaffected, some reduction in good practice is almost bound to occur. This may vary from the obvious to the more subtle. Workers may unwittingly mirror organisational processes by failing to listen, not attending to the user's concerns, becoming an adversary or being drawn into inappropriate or collusive relationships.

How can supervision help?

Fortunately, few organisations are outright 'red'. More often, organisations go through red and green phases and different parts of the organisation have different strengths and weaknesses. In all but the worst of organisational environments, frontline managers and supervisors have a remarkable ability to punch above their organisational weight. In doing so, good supervisors keep at bay the worst aspects of the organisation's functions and create a 'green space' where staff can continue to work well. What is noticeable about these supervisors is that they:

■ believe in the value and importance of their service

■ hold high professional standards

■ help staff understand broader policy and professional contexts

■ help staff identify and value their good practice

■ involve staff in problem solving, such as developing green cycle team strategies

■ connect with staff and their concerns

■ develop a strong team and learning ethos

■ model respectful behaviour to staff, service users and partners

■ show persistence and optimism in the face of difficulties

■ develop positive relationships with partners

■ make supervision a priority.

The key to supervisors maintaining a green space is the level of support that they receive. All of the issues discussed within this chapter are equally relevant to senior managers who supervise frontline supervisors. To expect supervisors to manage complex emotions without similar support themselves is unrealistic and organisations need to consider carefully the quality of supervision throughout the organisation. Frontline supervisors need to demand the same quality of supervision as they are expected to deliver. Support for supervisors is explored more fully in Chapter 8.

'The human encounter in the helping professions is inherently stressful. The stress aroused can be accommodated and used for the good of our clients. But our emotional responsiveness will wither if the human encounter cannot be contained within the institutions in which we work. By contrast, if we can maintain contact with the emotional reality of our clients and ourselves, then the human encounter can facilitate not only a healing experience, but also an enriching experience for them and for us.' (Tonnesmann (1979) in Hawkins & Shohet (1989))

References

Baumrind D (1978) Parental disciplinary patterns and social competence in children. *Youth and Society* **9** (3) 239–267.

Bourn D & Hafford-Letchfield T (2011) The role of social work professional supervision in conditions of uncertainty. *The International Journal of Knowledge, Culture and Change Management* **10** (9) 41–56.

Damasio A (2006) cited in Munro E (2007) *Effective Child Protection*. London: Sage.

Ekman P (1985) *Marketplace, Politics and Marriage*. New York, NY: Norton.

Gibbs J (2001) Maintaining frontline workers in child protection: a case for re-focusing supervision. *Child Abuse Review* **10** 323–335.

Goleman D, Boyatzis R & Mckee A (2002) *Primal Leadership: Realizing the power of emotional intelligence*. Boston, MA: Harvard Business School Press.

Howe D (2008) *The Emotionally Intelligent Social Worker*. Basingstoke: Palgrave Macmillan.

Hughes L & Pengelly P (1997) *Staff Supervision in a Turbulent World*. London: Jessica Kingsley.

Isen A (2000) Positive affect and decision making. In: M Lewis and J Haviland-Jones. *The Handbook of Emotions (2nd edition)*. Guildford Press: New York.

Lambley S & Marrable T (2013) *Practice Enquiry into Supervision in a Variety of Adult Care Settings where there are Health and Social Care Practitioners Working Together*. London: SCIE

Lexmond J & Reeves R (2009) *Building Character*. London: Demos.

Mayer JD & Salovey P (1997) What is emotional intelligence? In: P Salovey and D Sluyter (eds) *Emotional Development and Emotional Intelligence: Implications for educators* pp3–31. NY: Basic Books.

Menzies-Lyth L (1970) *The Functioning of Social Systems as a Defence Against Anxiety*. London: Tavistock Institute of Human Relations.

Morrison T (2007) Emotional intelligence, emotion and social work: context, characteristics, complications and contribution. *British Journal of Social Work* **37** (2) 245–263.

Richards J & Gross J (2000) Emotional regulation and memory: the cognitive costs of keeping one's cool. *Journal of Personality and Social Psychology* **79** pp410–424. Quoted in D Caruso and P Salovey (2004) *The Emotionally Intelligent Manager*. San Francisco, CA: Jossey-Bass.

Stanley J & Goddard C (2002) *In the Firing Line: Violence and power in child protection work*. Chichester: Wiley.

Tonnesmann M (1979) in Hawkins P & Shohet R (1989) *Supervision in the Helping Professions*. Buckingham: OU Press.

Wonnacott J (2012) *Mastering Social Work Supervision*. London: JKP.

Wells K (2004) *Emotional Intelligence as an Ability and its Relationship with Openness to Difference* (dissertation). San Diego, CA: Alliant International University.

Chapter 5: Supervising frontline practice: working with complexity

Whatever role a member of staff is carrying out within the human services, they will be working daily in situations where the outcomes of their actions are unlikely to be certain and there will be a variety of stakeholders with potentially differing views as to what good practice looks like. This, coupled with the possibility that the work will have personal resonances for the staff involved and may involve working with pain and distress, means that the supervision of any staff working directly with service users' needs to take account of the complexity of the task.

The work of Grint (2005) may be helpful here. Grint's work on problem solving describes problems as being either critical, tame or wicked.

- **Critical** – requires immediate intervention, needs an answer. Requires use of hierarchical power.

- **Tame** – encountered regularly, so have organisational procedures. Requires use of legitimate power.

- **Wicked** – The problem is ill-structured, with an evolving set of interlocking issues and constraints. There are so many factors and conditions, all embedded in a dynamic social context, that no two wicked problems are alike, and the solutions to them will always be custom designed and fitted. There may be no solutions, or there may be a host of potential solutions and another host that are never even thought of.

It is not too hard to see that although some problems in health and social care may be critical, most fall into the wicked category. However, despite this, for much of the early 21st century the approach has been based on a compliance model where practitioners (often driven by IT systems) are focused on meeting deadlines and targets rather than having the leeway to exercise professional judgement and be flexible in order to meet the needs of the individual. The underlying assumption with this approach is that most problems are 'tame' and can be managed solely via procedures and protocols. Supervision has therefore tended to follow suit with a focus on compliance, which research would suggest could set people up to fail (Manzoni & Barsoux, 1999). The set-up-to-fail syndrome is explored further in Chapter 6.

Grint goes on to explore what the best response might be to each type of problem.

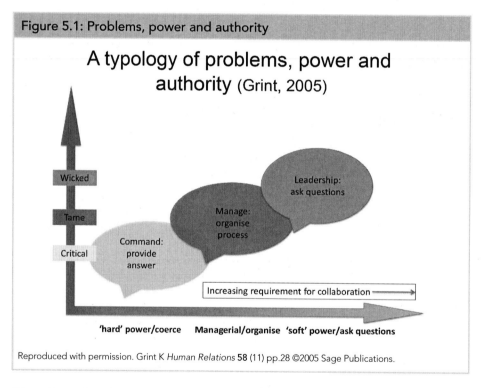

Figure 5.1: Problems, power and authority

Reproduced with permission. Grint K *Human Relations* **58** (11) pp.28 ©2005 Sage Publications.

If we recognise that most problems are 'wicked', this leads us a different style of supervision in line with that described by the supervision cycle. A key role for the supervisor is to develop their role as a leader of practice through asking questions which enable critical reflective practice and an exploration of the many interacting factors that will be influencing the work of their supervisee.

Crucial to this exploration is the role of the supervisor in promoting engagement with the stages of the supervision cycle which focus on reflection and analysis. The six stage cycle is an expansion of the supervision cycle and provides a framework for considering the various ways in which the supervisor can assist their supervisee to reflect on the underlying factors affecting practice, as well as using an analytical approach to deciding on future action.

The six stage cycle originates from unpublished training materials developed by Tony Morrison and subsequently used to train social workers across England as part of the Children's Workforce Development Council's training programmes (Morrison & Wonnacott, 2009). In its original form it focused on the supervision of assessment practice but, in recognition that assessment is a continuous process throughout all our work with service users, this model has now been developed as an approach which is relevant to the supervision of any frontline practice.

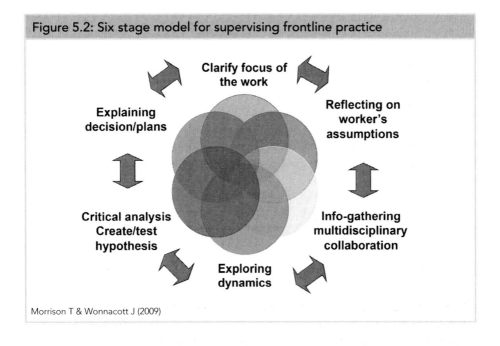

Figure 5.2: Six stage model for supervising frontline practice

Morrison T & Wonnacott J (2009)

This cycle describes six key elements in the effective supervision of practice. The interlocking circles show that this is a continuous and cyclical process rather than a linear one. Actions or responses in one area can trigger a reaction in any or all of the others. As an expansion of the supervisory cycle (experience, reflection, analysis and planning), it includes the same four stages, but in a slightly different order. The cycle starts not with experience (the information gathering stage) but with clarifying the purpose and focus of the work with the service user. This is one of the new elements. This cycle also divides reflection into two sections; preparatory reflection on the worker's initial assumptions and views about the case is separated from an exploration of the worker–service user relationship. The analysis and planning elements are the same as for the four-stage cycle.

The theory driving the development of the cycle is our understanding from research and practice of the way in which intuition, assumptions and biases will be important in driving practice responses. This, combined with information that may be open to interpretation and the uniqueness of each individual situation, means that exercising professional judgement is not an exact science but will be influenced by a range of factors. If we are to move from an over-reliance on procedures and process to a more balanced position where appropriate use of professional judgement is supported, the role and skill of the supervisor in working with the less tangible aspects of practice becomes even more crucial. In addition, a focus on the dynamics of relationships with service users and across the professional network is crucial to maximising the way in which supervision can positively impact on all the stakeholders.

Biases, assumptions and intuition

Supervision needs to start from the premise that both supervisor and supervisee will be bringing their own biases and assumptions to the table and it is crucial that supervisors create an environment where this is to be expected rather than seen as any weakness on the part of the supervisee. For example, a non-disabled person working with disabled people will bring their own culturally determined biases which have been influenced by the culture within which they have been brought up. A supervisee working with a family where alcohol misuse is an issue will be influenced by their own attitude to and experience of alcohol and all professionals are likely to be influenced by their most relevant experience of working with a similar case. These biases will affect practice from the beginning of any work they carry out and this is why the six stage cycle encourages reflection on assumptions *before* and *after* the information gathering stage. Munro (2008) noted that workers are liable to focus on a restricted range of evidence and use one of several techniques for discounting evidence that challenges their ideas. These techniques are:

- avoidance
- forgetting
- rejecting
- reinterpreting.

Workers, particularly those working in the field of child protection, have been criticised for their failure to pick up on crucial information in their work with families and maintain a 'respectful uncertainty' in their work. While undoubtedly recognising anxiety is crucial here (see Chapter 4) so also is the need to explore the underpinning assumptions and potential for bias. Supervisors play an important role in facilitating this.

The role of intuition

Linked to the above is recognition of the role of intuition and the importance of supervision allowing exploration of any 'gut feelings' experienced by the supervisee as well as integrating these intuitive responses with the analytical thinking needed to inform professional judgements and decisions.

Intuitive thinking is a largely unconscious process where we integrate a large amount of information to produce a judgement in a relatively effortless way, based on identifying patterns, feelings and images based on our previous experience. Gigerenza (2007) argues that intuition is best seen as an alternative method of reasoning that has evolved as we adapt to our environment:

'Gut feelings are therefore, neither impeccable nor stupid. They take advantage of the evolved capacities of the brain and are based on rules of thumb that enable us to act fast and with astonishing accuracy.' (Gigerenza, 2007 quoted in Munro, 2008, p.11)

By contrast, Munro (2008) describes analytic thinking as:

'*conscious and controlled using formal reasoning and explicit data and rules to deliberate and compute a conclusion. It is restricted by memory and processing capacity, time-consuming, and effortful. It develops with age and is vulnerable to the aging process.*' (p11)

Munro's central point is that professionals need to use both intuitive and analytic methods of thinking and decision making. The skill is to know when to use which method, as they each have benefits and limitations as outlined in **Table 5.1: Pros and cons of intuitive and analytic decisions**.

Table 5.1: Pros and cons of intuitive and analytic decisions

Benefits of intuitive model	Disadvantages	Benefits of analytic method	Disadvantages
Can process speedily, especially in conditions of urgency	Over confidence in 'my gut feeling' leads to poor judgements	Good when a complex or contested decision is required	Takes time and effort
Better for immediate/short-term decisions	Relies on personal experience	Ensures systematic data collection and analysis	Requires training
Validates emotions and hunches as important information	Limited by information capacity of short-term memory	Maximises options and alternatives	
Values contribution regardless of status or experience	Short-term focus results in lack of contingency plans	Based on formal probability theory	Can be hard to engage busy practitioners and manager
Can be very accurate for modest effort	Generates low-level theory with limited application	Can generate higher level theory with wider application	Can be used to bolster elitist/expert attitudes
Values life experience and practice wisdom	We seek to confirm own beliefs despite the evidence	Supports public explanation of decision	Can be manipulated to justify decisions as scientific or objective

Supervisors need to be aware of these advantages and disadvantages and work together with their supervisees to integrate both approaches in their work.

The nature of information: working with discrepancy

The nature and presentation of information in any field of social care is rarely straightforward. In the field of safeguarding children and adults, it can be particularly complex and ambiguous due to professional and inter-agency anxiety, fear of getting it wrong and limited skills in communicating effectively with service users, particularly children and those with communication differences. In other words, information in this field rarely comes with clarity about what it is, how it has been obtained and what it means.

It is the task of practitioners, supervisors and multidisciplinary planning meetings to share, sift, search for and determine how important their information is. It is through this process that raw data (facts, feelings and beliefs) can be transformed into useful intelligence. Often, one piece of the jigsaw only makes sense when fitted together with the other pieces.

Five types of discrepancy

One way to think about this issue is the idea of discrepancy, namely when one piece of information does not fit another piece.

Five types of discrepancy that can occur in an inter-agency environment

1. Informational: there is contradictory information from different agencies.

2. Interpretative: different conclusions are drawn from the same information by different people.

3. Interactive: the intentions of the service user and others in their network are contradicted by actions.

4. Incongruent: the way in which people talk about another person is inconsistent, contradictory or incoherent.

5. Instinctual: gut feelings indicate that something is wrong but they cannot specify what this is.

Indications or clues about the existence of such discrepancies can occur at organisational, inter-agency, service user and practitioner levels.

Figure 5.3: Examples of discrepancy shows some examples.

Figure 5.3: Examples of discrepancy

Organisational clues

- Organisational/team mythology exists about 'this service user and/ or family is...'
- Negative stereotypes about other agencies exist so their information is discounted.
- Sudden changes about view of risk not explained.
- Sudden changes of plan not explained.

Worker clues

- Gut feelings say something is wrong.
- Worker does not ask difficult questions.
- Analysis does not account for facts/history.
- Proposed plan does not address issues identified in the assessment.
- Practitioner is working much harder than others in the system, including relevant family, to effect change.
- The service user's story is missing.

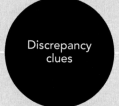

Discrepancy clues

Interagency clues

- Agencies have conflicting views of the family/risk.
- Agencies have strong views but offer ambiguous/limited evidence.
- Some agencies unwilling to share information.
- Pressure to agree suppresses permission to question.

Family/service user clues

- Intentions not supported by actions.
- One family members account conflicts with another.
- Inconsistencies/lack of coherence in description of issues.
- Optimism involves denial of difficulties.
- Co-operation is only on the family/ servicer user's terms.
- Team working enhanced.

At the heart of these discrepancies are tensions between belief and behaviour, or between conviction and evidence.

Figure 5.4: The discrepancy matrix shows how different types of evidence and belief can produce four different types of information: ambiguous, missing, assumption-led or coherent information.

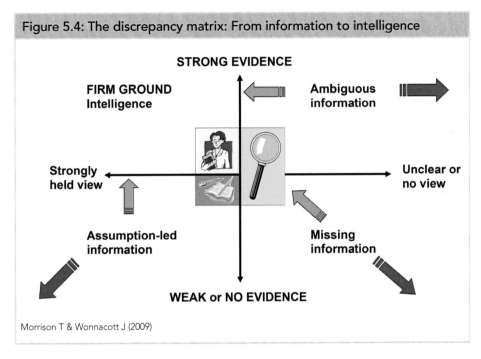

Figure 5.4: The discrepancy matrix: From information to intelligence

STRONG EVIDENCE

FIRM GROUND
Intelligence

Ambiguous
information

Strongly
held view

Unclear or
no view

Assumption-led
information

Missing
information

WEAK or NO EVIDENCE

Morrison T & Wonnacott J (2009)

The arrows indicate the need to inquire further and dig deeper to decide whether the information is useful and relevant. If so, it moves towards coherent information (green arrow). Alternatively, testing the information may eliminate it, either as irrelevant or as ungrounded (red arrow).

Supervision, represented by scrutiny (magnifying glass), the face-to-face discussion and the recording of information, is fundamental in helping the worker sift and test the information. This can lead to highlighting and exploring discrepancies in information, and deciding whether further inquiries are needed to clarify whether the information is valuable.

This approach starts from the viewpoint that raw information is almost always complex and problematic. However, good supervision can help to test and explore assumptions, ambiguities or gaps in information, ensuring that analysis and planning are on solid foundations.

Information gathering and multidisciplinary collaboration

The supervisor's role here falls into five main areas:

1. Guiding the worker about key information that needs to be gathered and used to inform their practice.

2. Identifying potential sources of information and how to access these.

3. Communicating effectively with other agencies who are involved with the service user.

4. Evaluating the quality of information.

5. Helping the worker organise and record the information they have collected.

Depending on the nature of the setting within which the supervisee is working, various techniques might be used to gather information as work progresses. For example:

- the development of a chronology in order to understand the history of previous involvement between the organisation and the service user

- the construction of a genogram with the service user(s) in order to understand their family history and context

- the development of an ecomap – ie. a diagram showing the professional network working with the service user and relationship between its members.

At the heart of all these approaches is the capacity of the worker to engage with the service user and other professionals in order to gather and sift relevant information.

Information is not an objective collection of data; it is determined by the nature of the dialogue between the supervisor and worker. However, because

Developing and Supporting Effective Staff Supervision: A reader © Pavilion Publishing and Media Ltd and its licensors 2014.

of the difference in power and experience of the two parties, the focus of the supervisor's questions about the information obtained by the worker will largely decide what the worker tells the supervisor. This means that if the supervisor does not ask about a certain area, the information may be lost. The worker quickly learns what information their supervisor usually favours, which may impact on both the type of information the worker then seeks from the service user and how they seek it. This is why it is so important that the supervisor accesses all six parts of the supervision of frontline practice cycle.

Exploring dynamics within a multidisciplinary network

In addition, multidisciplinary information cannot be taken at face value, so the supervisor needs to help the worker evaluate the content; the meaning of information is rarely self-explanatory, whether it is coming from family members, other agencies, and your own organisation or from the practitioner. Reder and Duncan (2003) argue that supervision is an ideal opportunity for practitioners to review how they communicate with others by thinking systemically – bearing in mind other professionals who are involved in the case.

Key messages from Reder and Duncan (2003) are:

- communication and co-ordination are distinct activities; co-ordination is an inter-agency context, within which communication can occur

- communication is the process by which information is transferred from one person to another *and is understood* by them

- information includes both factual information and also feelings, attitudes and desires

- when one person transfers a message to another, a process of meta communication (communication about the communication) takes place. This relates to the way in which non-verbal components such as tone and emotional content either reinforce the message, or qualify it. It is therefore imperative to explore not only whether communication happened but the meaning ascribed to the communication by both parties

- it is the responsibility of both the message giver and receiver to ensure that their communication is being understood by the other – monitoring mutual understanding

- messages given thoughtlessly and without purpose are likely to get 'lost' in transmission

- personal and interpersonal factors will influence the outcome of an episode of communication, for example:
  - feelings about the other person or organisation
  - anxieties and workload pressures
  - personal beliefs and prejudices
  - organisational context.

Effective supervision will move beyond an approach which ensures that communication happened, to collaborating with the supervisee in interrogating the meaning of the communication and hence its effectiveness.

Supervision and the meaning of communication

- *Acknowledgement that communication occurred*

  - Did you telephone the GP?
  - So we received another referral about Sam...

- *Description of the detail of the communication*

  - What did you ask? What was their response?
  - How was the referral made? What were the concerns this time?

- *Exploration of feelings and emotions within the communication*

  - Have you had previous contact with that particular professional?
  - What happened then, and how did you feel about it?
  - How do you feel about what the other feels about you?
  - How do you feel about the information/response?

- *Understanding the meaning of the communication*

  - How far has the quality or content of the communication between you been affected by previous experiences or current expectations?
  - How might they perceive your role?
  - Are there any issues of power and hierarchy that may have affected the communication?

- *Exploring the implications of the communication*

  - What further questions do we need to ask?
  - What are the implications of this communication for our next steps?

Dynamics within groups – understanding 'groupthink'

Workers will often be working with groups both within and across professional boundaries and many crucial judgements and decisions are made within a group context. Time is needed in supervision to explore the way group process will influence decision making.

Janis (1982) coined the term 'groupthink' to explain the biases within groups that may lead to distorted reasoning. Groupthink involves a desire to avoid conflict and results in a reluctance to challenge the group consensus. Group judgement and decision making are therefore vulnerable to the two biases of avoiding conflicting views and tending towards consensus around an extreme position. Janis proposed measures to avoid groupthink which include group members discussing the group's deliberations with trusted associates and reporting these discussions to the group. Supervision can fulfil this role.

Exploring the dynamics between supervisee and service users

The main tasks for the supervisor here are:

- to monitor the quality of the worker's relationships and interactions with service users

- to help the worker reflect on these interactions

- to identify and assist the worker with the emotional impact of the case and its effect on their work.

Attitudes, assumptions and the interpretation of information are strongly linked to interactions, relationships and emotions, which is why it is vital that the emotional aspects of the work are brought into the supervision process. There are three reasons for this.

Firstly, emotions lie at the heart of the gut feelings and intuitive judgements that play such a significant role in professional analysis. If these reactions can't be discussed and remain suppressed, this can undermine the work with service users. It may also result in the supervisor missing vital clues about risks to adults and children which are picked up subconsciously in the worker's own responses to family dynamics. Inexperienced workers in particular can be drawn into such dynamics, which may lead to them becoming enmeshed with the family, unable to see the dangers for vulnerable members and drawn into an alliance with powerful or intimidating family members. Supervisors need to keep a watchful eye out for any evidence that the worker appears to be over-identifying with a particular family member, or acting out one family member's script.

Secondly, the quality of relationships between family members and workers is crucial to the outcome of the work. In order to create a climate where service users and their families can engage with the process and be open about problems, the relationship skills of the worker are essential. The quality of the social worker's relationships also has a big impact on the likelihood of change. Therefore, one of the main tasks of the supervisor is to monitor the worker–service users/family relationship and to be aware of signs of confusion, conflict, coldness, collusion or fear. These might be picked up in a number of ways:

- noticing how the worker talks about different family members, in particular vulnerable children and adults
- noticing how the worker talks about different sorts of risks and harm
- noticing how the worker talks about service users/family members from different cultures
- being alert to what the worker does NOT talk about
- noting discrepancies in the worker's or other's accounts
- comparing the way that co-workers react to service users
- reading reports and noting the language used by the worker
- observing the worker's interaction with the service user/family
- asking the worker to reflect on their interactions.

Lastly, the needs, perceptions and concerns of vulnerable service users are often brought to the surface by exploring feelings. This is especially in the case of children or others with communication differences. Consider how these questions can bring the service user into the supervision process.

- If the service user could tell the story of the last three months of their life, what do you think they would say and what would be their strongest feelings?

- How does the service user's story support or challenge the story of others in their network?

- How much do you know about what he/she feels?

- If the service user was given a magic wand and invited to change one thing about their life, what do you think they would choose?

Critical analysis

At this stage the supervisor will be working with their supervisee to integrate their intuitive responses with analytical reasoning in order to form a view about the meaning of information including risks, strengths, service user capacities and vulnerabilities. This stage will involve an exploration of the impact of all of these factors for future work and make the link between current experience, known information and decisions and plans.

The main tasks for the supervisor are:

- to ensure the worker has explored how others, especially service users, see issues/problems and their impact

- to help the worker express their understanding of what is happening and consider alternative possible explanations

- to identify what further information is required at this stage of the work

- to help the worker develop an evidence-based understanding of their work including using information from practice, personal experience, theory and research

- family members' explanations

- social workers' understandings gained from practice and personal experience

- research knowledge

- formal theories.

Too often this stage of the supervision process is weak, and within children's services there has been criticism of the lack of analytical recording within both case records and supervision notes. Training supervisors has, however, shown that the analytical process can be helped by the use of tools to support analysis. Any tool that transfers information and interpretation from inside the worker's head to an external description of events, patterns and possible explanations will improve the quality of analysis. It will also help the worker and supervisor explore together the information and its interpretation. Tools will vary depending upon the working context but several of the tools that can assist information gathering, such as genograms and ecomaps, can also assist analysis. Other tools, such as frameworks for analysing risk applied to a particular case, assessing motivation to change (Morrison, 2010) and decision trees, may also be helpful.

Decision and plans

The six stage cycle refers to this as 'explaining decisions and plans'. All the factors explored in relation to the four stage supervision cycle apply here, with the addition that frontline practice should be underpinned by the capacity to be clear both with the service user and others as to why a certain course of action is being taken. If the previous stages of the cycle have been used well in supervision, by this point workers should be able to articulate why they are doing what they are doing.

Questions to support the use of the six stage cycle

The following questions should not be used as a checklist but they do provide a guide for supervisors supervising practice on the front line.

1. **Clarifying the focus of the work**

■ What is the task in this situation?

■ What is the purpose of the task?

■ Are there any frameworks and protocols that should be informing the work?

■ Which aspects of the work will be more challenging for you?

- What are the possible outcomes?

- What are the limits to the work you are involved with at present?

- What support and guidance do you need from your supervisor?

2. **Initial views, assumptions and knowledge base**

- What questions do you have about this piece of work?

- List three assumptions you might have formed on the basis of the information in this case.

- If you had any bias in this case, what would it be?

- What beliefs do professionals already have about this family/person?

- What cultural or gender issues might arise?

- What knowledge do you bring to this case? Where does it come from?

- Are there gaps in your knowledge?

- What previous experience do you have of similar work? How do you think that might influence your approach?

- What was the outcome last time you worked with a similar situation?

- What questions/feelings might the user have about the work you are doing with them?

3. **Information gathering**

- What are the key pieces of information you need at the moment?

- What do we already know?

- What don't we know?

- Where and who are the agency sources for this information?

- Who knows the family/person best?

- Which other agencies/services need to be involved at the moment?

- How might other agencies see your role in this family?

- Is any agency likely to be difficult to engage? How might we address this?

- Would there be any benefit in co-working?

- What contact and information from other agencies do you need?

- Which family members and friends need to be involved currently?

- How are you recording information?

- What discrepancies in information exist?

- How do we test or resolve these?

- What information do we need from other agencies that we still do not have?

4. **Worker–service user dynamics**

- How would you describe your approach to this work?

- What would I notice about it?

- How do you think Mrs X would describe your approach and style? If you had to describe the dynamics between you and the family/individual, would it be more like 'cat and mouse', 'pulling teeth', 'a shared voyage of discovery', 'just another piece of work' or something else?

- How does your interaction with the service user help/hinder the work?

- What is easy/hard to talk about in relation to this work?

- What, if any, contradictory/confusing signals have you picked up in the interaction between family members and yourself/other professionals?

- Who or what does this piece of work remind you of?

- What has most surprised/concerned you about the family/person?

- What is your gut reaction about this family/individual? Where does this come from?

5. **Worker's analysis**

- What is becoming clearer? What is becoming less clear? What is unknown?

- What positive or concerning patterns are emerging in this work?

- How long-standing are these patterns?

- To what extent does the information gathered confirm or challenge your initial impressions?

- What pieces of information are still not making sense or are ambiguous?

- How can we clarify these?

- How does the information gathered most likely explain the causes and consequences of any current concerns?

- What alternative explanations need to be considered?

- How do other agencies understand the situation? What are their concerns?

- What is the user's explanation for the situation they are in?

- What do you think is the meaning of this situation to them?

- What risk and protective factors exist in this case?

- What might other agencies/the service users make of how we are thinking about this case currently?

- How can we test which explanation is likely to be more robust?

- What knowledge, theory, research, values and experience can help explain this situation and how it might develop?

- What specific outcomes for the service user do we need to be seeing in order to address the issues identified?

- If there is no professional intervention, will things be better, worse or the same in six months' time? Think about the different family members involved.

6. Decisions and plans

- What decisions do we need to make at this point?

- What options are there?

- To what extent do we have the information to make a decision at this point?

- What might be the pros and cons of different decisions? Who gains and who loses?

- What is negotiable and non-negotiable about this situation in relation to our organisation's duties and responsibilities?

- To what extent is there agreement between agencies about the issues in this case?

- What would the best possible outcome look like for the service user?

- What services or interventions are required to achieve this outcome?

- What specific outcomes have been or need to be identified in the plan for the child/parents?

- How clear are your/others' roles and specific tasks in helping these outcomes become a reality?

- What is motivating the service user/family to work with you?

- How does the plan provide for monitoring and review against the intended outcomes?

- What is the contingency plan if these aren't achieved?

- How clear are you about the framework for recording this piece of work?

- Where would it be helpful to record the underpinning theory/research that is informing your decisions?

- How fair, clear, balanced and evidence-based is your recording? Is it clear how the decision/recommendation was arrived at?

- What is your plan for sharing your thinking and any written report with family members?

References

Gigerenza G (2007) in Munro E (2008) *Effective Child Protection*. London: Sage.

Grint K (2005) Problems, problems, problems: the social construction of 'leadership'. *Human Relations* **58** (11) 1467–1494.

Janis I (1982) *Groupthink: Psychological studies of policy decisions and fiascos*. Boston, MA: Houghton Mifflin.

Manzoni J-F & Barsoux J-L (1999) 'The Set-Up-to-Fail Syndrome' in *Harvard Business Review on Managing People*. Harvard Business School Press.

Morrison T & Wonnacott J (2009) Unpublished training materials.

Morrison T (2010) The strategic leadership of complex practice. *Child Abuse Review* **19** 312–329.

Munro E (2008) *Effective Child Protection* (2nd edition). London: Sage.

Reder P & Duncan S (2003) *Beyond Blame: Child abuse tragedies revisited*. London: Routledge.

Chapter 6: Supervising to improve performance

One of the key roles of the supervisor, whether or not they are the manager of the supervisee, is to remain focused on improving outcomes for service users through developing practice and improving performance. At times this will involve identifying areas of the work where the supervisee is struggling and addressing performance issues; an area of supervision practice that can feel uncomfortable and challenging. All too often, low-level concerns are just ignored. This not only reduces the quality of service but also stunts the worker's own development and potentially stores up more serious problems for the future. In many cases, this is because the organisation's performance management systems and managerial support for supervisors haven't been good enough. As a result, supervisors' own confidence to address such issues declines, and there is an increased tolerance towards concerning behaviour and practice, all of which can also be seen in worker/service user relationships. This chapter focuses on frameworks and strategies to prevent this happening, through taking a positive approach to improving performance underpinned by the following beliefs.

- Supervision is an authority relationship within which the supervisor has responsibility to work with the supervisee to improve practice.

- The authority of the supervisor depends more on the way they behave than their job description.

- Staff will work best when expectations are clear.

- Staff who get stuck can be helped.

- Supervisors will be most effective if they understand why supervisees are stuck and the function of their blocks.

- Organisations have a responsibility to provide a clear framework for addressing performance issues.

- An essential component of the supervisory relationship is giving feedback on the worker's strengths.

- Failure to prevent underperformance benefits no one.

Working to improve performance can be described along a continuum from creating the conditions whereby staff can succeed, through to HR action (Wonnacott, 2012).

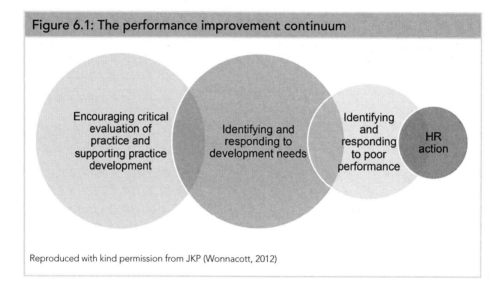

Figure 6.1: The performance improvement continuum

Encouraging critical evaluation of practice and supporting practice development

Identifying and responding to development needs

Identifying and responding to poor performance

HR action

Reproduced with kind permission from JKP (Wonnacott, 2012)

This continuum highlights the need for supervisors to work at many different levels, always engaging proactively in discussions about the quality of day-to-day practice activity. Appropriate use of their 'professional authority' (Hughes & Pengelly, 1997) and role as a leader of practice is an important aspect of their supervisory work. This was confirmed by the research review (Carpenter *et al*, 2012) and SCIE practice enquiry into the components of effective supervision (Lambley & Marrable, 2013), which noted the importance of having supervisors who are up-to-date in their clinical expertise and are able to provide tangible work-related guidance (task assistance) and feedback to their supervisees.

Figure 6.2: Managing performance through leadership (Wonnacott, 2012) sets this within a framework which recognises the importance of the supervisor in knowing what good practice looks like and establishing a culture and environment within which their supervisees can practice effectively. Depending on their place within the organisation, this may involve the supervisor in liaising with others and alerting more senior managers to any factors that are inhibiting good practice, as well as establishing team cultures where an atmosphere of mutual support and opportunities for reflection make success more likely. Building on this, the effective supervisor will recognise good practice and encourage their own supervisees and others in the team to learn from what works well. It is within this context of openness and honesty that performance concerns can be identified and managed, action taken to improve practice and, in a minority of situations, formal intervention can be taken.

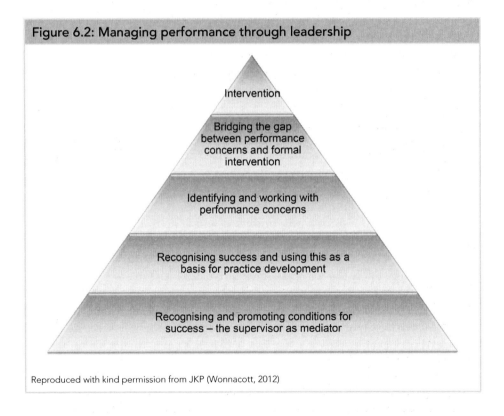

Figure 6.2: Managing performance through leadership

Intervention

Bridging the gap between performance concerns and formal intervention

Identifying and working with performance concerns

Recognising success and using this as a basis for practice development

Recognising and promoting conditions for success – the supervisor as mediator

Reproduced with kind permission from JKP (Wonnacott, 2012)

Positive expectations perspective

The approach outlined previously can be described as one which is based on 'positive expectations'. The positive expectations approach states that:

- staff want to do a good job
- no one wants to be ineffective
- staff work best when they are clear about their role and responsibility
- people can and will try to change if it makes sense to them
- performance can be improved if weaknesses are identified and worked on
- being clear what good work looks like helps people change
- it is the behaviour and not the personality that needs to change
- healthy disagreement creates the conditions for change
- agreed action on improving performance enhances commitment and trust.

Appreciative enquiry

Appreciative enquiry (Cooperrider *et al*, 2008) is one theoretical perspective and practice tool which may help supervisors create a culture of positive expectations and build on practice success. It is based on the premise that 'organisations change in the direction in which they inquire'. An organisation which inquires into problems will keep finding problems, but if an organisation attempts to appreciate what is best in itself, it will discover more and more good. In practical terms it provides another lens through which to think about the way questions are asked within supervision.

By using an appreciative enquiry approach to questioning within supervision, the supervisor can move beyond a culture which focuses on mistakes to one where the worker can risk being open about their practice since as much (if not more) attention is paid to learning from success as exploring difficulties.

Using this approach, the supervisor may ask the following:

- Tell me about a time when you were working with a service user who did not want to engage with you but you turned it around.
  - What was the situation?
  - What were you feeling?
  - What did you say?
  - What did you do?
  - What happened to transform the situation?

- Tell me about the last time you felt really excited about a piece of work you did with a family. Describe it to me in detail.

- You told me last time that you really didn't want to take on this piece of work, but you did and it went well.
  - What conversations did you have with yourself before you started?
  - What support did you receive from others to help you do it?
  - What made it a success?

What shapes performance?

Creating the conditions for success, learning from success and identifying points where supervisees may struggle, requires supervisors to consider all the factors that might shape performance at a particular point in time. Rogers (1999) suggests that personal effectiveness or performance results from the fit between three factors.

1. The individual's values, experience, skills, personality, motivation and expectations.

2. The job role, demands, responsibilities, control and complexity.

3. The organisation's culture, systems, teams and services.

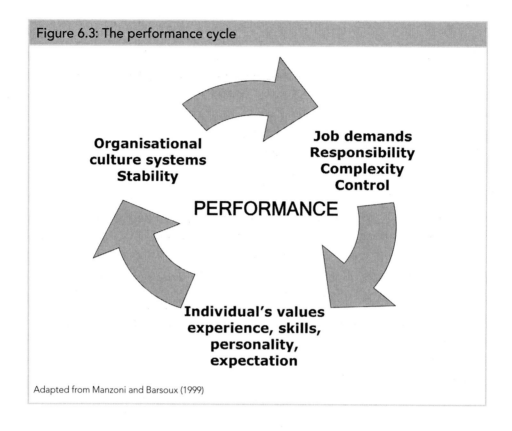

Figure 6.3: The performance cycle

Organisational culture systems Stability

Job demands Responsibility Complexity Control

PERFORMANCE

Individual's values experience, skills, personality, expectation

Adapted from Manzoni and Barsoux (1999)

Expectancy theory

Expectancy theory states that it is the anticipated satisfaction of a valued outcome that shapes behaviour towards that outcome. Motivation is explained in terms of two related factors: expectancy and instrumentality (Vroom, 1964).

1. Expectancy: 'Can I make X happen?' This is how far a person believes that behaving in a certain way will make something happen.

2. Instrumentality: 'If I do this, will it be worth it?' This is the perceived probability that making X happen will result in something worthwhile happening.

For example, a supervisor may identify that a supervisee has concerns about report writing. As we can see in **Figure 6.3**, the worker's expectations and motivation are influenced by the organisational environment and the nature of their job, and the social worker's perception of their ability to improve this will be related to a number of factors:

- clarity about organisational expectations and systems for report writing
- the nature and complexity of the report writing task
- the quality of the feedback process
- the worker's skills, professional values and standards of report writing
- the time and support to do the task.

The supervisor starts by providing specific feedback to the worker, and links this to organisational and professional expectations about report writing. The worker's difficulties with the task are explored and an improvement plan is drawn up. The supervisor provides assistance, such as training about report writing, and some protected report writing time. As a result, the worker's motivation improves, and their expectation that they will be able to improve their report writing increases, however, the chain can be broken at any point if, for instance:

- there are no standards about report writing
- no examples of good reports are provided
- the feedback from the supervisor is poorly delivered
- no specific improvement targets or plans are set.

Factors affecting performance

The above example highlights the importance of thinking about all the factors that might be affecting performance at a given time. They will be different for each individual and although **Figure 6.4: Factors contributing to underperformance** sets out possible issues to consider, the skill of the supervisor lies in working together with their supervisee to understand the impact of the various factors and crucially whether as a supervisor they are contributing to the problem.

Figure 6.4: Factors contributing to underperformance

Organisational factors

Unclear agency standards/policies

Inappropriate recruitment

Weak performance management

Rigid or inconsistent management practice

Inadequate HR support

Culture of no consequences

Poor/no supervision

Service under-capacity and/or instability

Ambiguous role/job design

Inappropriate or unmanageable workload

Systems failings (eg. inadequate IT)

Individual factors

Stress/major life event

Ill health/trauma

Lack of social support

Low emotional IQ

Weak self-regulation

Inflexibility

High anxiety

Limited cognitive skills

Limited written skills

Limited analysis skills

Inappropriate values

Language difficulties

Cultural conflicts

Underperformance

Inter-agency factors

eg. where workers are located in integrated settings or M/D team settings

Worker unclear on role

Governance arrangements unclear

Conflicting performance systems

Strained agency relationships

Poor M/D communication

Worker's role not understood

Role not valued by colleagues

Required to do inappropriate tasks

Conflicting value base

Professional factors

Inadequate knowledge and skills

Inadequate induction to the post

Inadequate training

Role/skill/aptitude mismatch

Change in working conditions

Emotional impact of the work

Complex/unpredictable service-user problems

Values conflict with organisation

Professional isolation

Disaffection with job/agency role

Morrison T (2009)

Understanding the factors that might be influencing performance will also help the supervisor to understand whether the problem is a capability problem (cannot) or a disinclination (will not) problem.

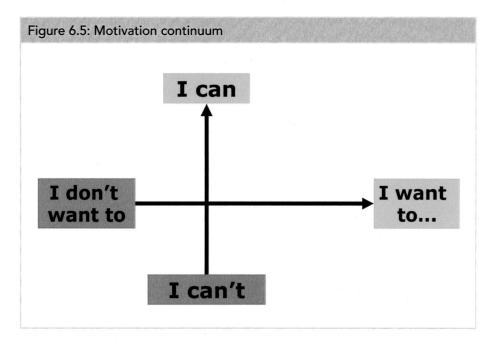

Figure 6.5: Motivation continuum

Sometimes it can be hard to separate capability from disinclination, since 'I can't' can be used to mask 'I won't' and vice-versa. Willingness to improve behaviour is partly related to confidence, not only within the worker, but from the supervisor. What is crucial is that the supervisor works with the supervisee to understand the difference, otherwise there is the possibility that in attempting to work with performance concerns they might set their supervisee up to fail. This analysis will need to include consideration not only of any organisational, professional and individual factors, but also whether the supervisor has unwittingly contributed to the concern.

The set-up-to-fail syndrome

Research by Manzoni and Barsoux (1999) suggests that it is often managers themselves who are unwittingly responsible for their employees' under-performance. The 'set-up-to-fail' syndrome typically occurs through the over-reaction of a supervisor to a low-level 'mistake' or 'failing' by the worker. This triggers the supervisor into over-managing the worker by being directive and interfering. The worker then feels that they are being unfairly judged and that the supervisor is making little attempt to understand what led to the failure.

As a result of this, the worker rapidly loses confidence and starts to withdraw from the supervisor (see **Figure 6.6: Set-up-to-fail syndrome**). After all, why would the worker wish to be exposed to further criticism? On top of this, the staff member may feel they're no longer part of the supervisor's 'in-group' and feel powerless within the supervisory relationship. One danger within a social care environment is that the worker may compensate by reasserting their power with service users, which inevitably results in the service user losing trust in the worker, which further vindicates the supervisor's original judgement.

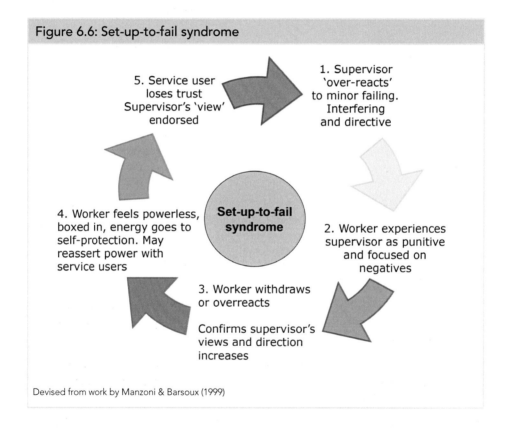

Figure 6.6: Set-up-to-fail syndrome

5. Service user loses trust Supervisor's 'view' endorsed

1. Supervisor 'over-reacts' to minor failing. Interfering and directive

Set-up-to-fail syndrome

4. Worker feels powerless, boxed in, energy goes to self-protection. May reassert power with service users

2. Worker experiences supervisor as punitive and focused on negatives

3. Worker withdraws or overreacts

Confirms supervisor's views and direction increases

Devised from work by Manzoni & Barsoux (1999)

In addition to describing this cycle, Manzoni and Barsoux (1999) also suggest that a large proportion of managers tend to treat stronger and weaker performers differently, resulting in an 'in versus out crowd' dynamic.

Table 6.1: The 'in' crowd and 'out' crowd	
The supervisor's 'in crowd'	The supervisor's 'out crowd'
Manager's behaviour towards stronger performers	**Manager's behaviour towards weaker performers**
Discusses the task, offering more freedom for the worker to decide the approach	Directive and detailed about the task and how it should be done
Lapses created as learning opportunities	Lapses treated as 'mistakes'
High availability – 'let me know if I can help'	Low availability or on manager's terms only – 'I need to see you when…'
Open to worker's suggestions, consults worker on their ideas	Little interest in worker's suggestions, or dismisses them
Praises worker for work well done	Focuses on what the worker has done poorly
Willing to defer to worker in disagreements	Imposes own views in disagreements

Adapted from Manzoni and Barsoux (1999)

In order to break this cycle, Manzoni and Barsoux (1999) suggest that supervisors need to:

■ create the right context for discussion – it is here that the time spent developing an effective supervisory relationship and including a quality agreement will pay off

■ agree together evidence-based symptoms of the problem – ie. do we both understand that performance could improve, and in what way?

■ arrive at a common understanding of what might be causing weak performance – ie. the factors that might be affecting work as explored earlier in this chapter

■ agree what future performance should look like (performance objectives) and how the supervisor can support the worker in achieving these (relationship objectives)

■ agree future communication methods – this might include asking for help early on, using ad hoc supervision etc.

Too often, the focus is solely on performance objectives without any fundamental agreement that there is a problem with practice in the first place and/or the factors affecting performance. If from the worker's perspective, the way they have written a report is quite acceptable whereas the supervisor feels it is not adequate, or the supervisee feels there has not been time to do a good job but the supervisor feels it is a lack of skill, it is unlikely that there will be any real engagement in working together to improve practice. Nothing is likely to be effective if the relationship is problematic and a focus on how to make this most effective is an essential element of breaking this cycle. Reviewing the supervision agreement at this point may be a useful approach.

The blocked cycle

Another way of thinking about under-performance and developing improvement strategies is under-performance as a response to an external stress. This can be anxiety, conflict, work overload, or role confusion, which results in the worker becoming 'stuck' and 'blocked', either temporarily or more widely. Recalling the supervisory cycle of experience, reflection, analysis and action, it is possible to see what happens when, instead of workers accessing all parts of the cycle, the worker gets stuck at one or more points. It is also possible to see how being 'stuck' at any of these points becomes self-protective for an anxious or overwhelmed worker.

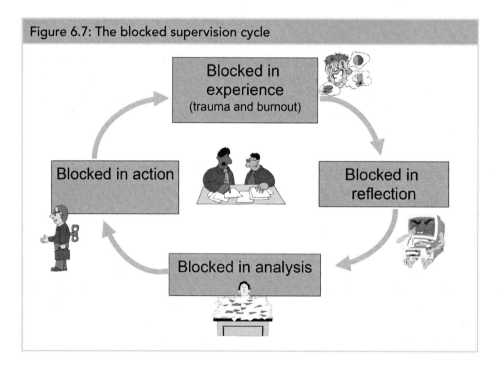

Figure 6.7: The blocked supervision cycle

Blocked in experience (trauma and burnout)

Blocked in action

Blocked in reflection

Blocked in analysis

The four stages of the cycle are described as follows.

Stuck in feelings

Instead of accessing and using feelings productively, the worker becomes stuck or mired in feelings, unable to think, analyse or plan clearly. This results in task delay and avoidance and leads to becoming much less productive. Focusing solely on feelings is self-protective for the worker because they become disengaged from observation and thinking and this reduces the amount of information they have to deal with. In doing so the worker's engagement with other perspectives, such as those of the service user, the organisation or other agencies is also reduced so that the worker becomes self-preoccupied (ie. 'it's all about me!'). In addition, the worker's high anxiety results in them seeking constant support from their supervisor and colleagues to complete simple tasks, thereby gaining considerable attention for their plight. The worker's 'vulnerability' in turn makes it harder for the supervisor to insist on tasks being completed, and for the worker to carry an equitable workload.

Stuck in analysis

Here the worker becomes narrow, inflexible and judgemental in their practice, unable to access feelings. The worker retreats to a bureaucratic mode of functioning, in which the outcomes seem almost pre-determined by the worker – (ie. 'it's one of these...'). While on the surface this may have the appearance of an efficient and productive performance by a worker who demands little of the supervisor, it is at the expense of real engagement with the service user, careful assessment and responsive planning. By avoiding feelings, resorting to procedural or 'checklist' responses, the worker regains a sense of control, safety and predictability and reduces the burden of professional responsibility and personal vulnerability.

Stuck in 'being busy'

Although excessive demands may from time-to-time be a feature of all staff's working life, here 'being busy' and 'being seen to be busy' become functional for the worker. The pattern is one of rushing around doing things for and to their service users, in a dependency-creating and paternalistic manner. Caught up in 'rescuing' activity, they may miss what is important for the service user, or fail to address difficult issues with users, where to do so would create conflict and threaten their 'relationship'. Their 'busy-busy' and reactive style makes proper assessment very difficult. It also means the worker is unable to engage with more emotionally demanding or complex issues. It is often compounded by avoidance of supervision and lack of engagement with their team and colleagues such that they become 'maverick' and no longer reliably represent the organisation. By creating dependency relationships, staying busy, not pausing to feel or think, the worker defines their role in a way that offers them a sense of public purpose and personal reward, while avoiding engagement with the real needs of their service users or the requirements of their organisation.

Stuck in experience

This describes situations in which the individual is overwhelmed by work demands or by the dynamics of a toxic work setting – recall the red cycle (see Chapter 4). In response, the worker turns down the volume controls of feeling, thinking and action due to their physical and emotional exhaustion. Another explanation is that this is a reaction to a traumatic experience. Sometimes such a response may occur in the context of a relatively minor work event, but one which triggers the memory of an earlier unresolved experience. Alternatively, the reaction occurs at a time when the worker is facing other stresses, perhaps at home. Either way, the result is professional paralysis and personal distress. To protect him or herself against the loss of control, confidence and competence, the worker retreats from engagement both with the external world and their own distressed state. By doing so, the individual gains physical and mental respite, and the reduction of exposure to potentially overwhelming demands.

The function of the blocked learning/performance cycle

This concept of the blocked cycle is one in which under-performance is seen as a response to anxiety, threat, unpredictability, and loss of control, confidence or competence. In order to restore a sense of safety, control, comfort, and predictability, the mind performs a number of unconscious, strategically protective operations. These are shown in **Figure 6.8: The blocked learning cycle – the mind's protective response**.

Figure 6.8: The blocked learning cycle – the mind's protective response

By reducing the amount of information the mind deals with, situations are simplified and complexity is avoided…

…which reduces awareness of demands, emotions, and differing perspectives…

…which leads to minimisation of roles, responsibility and accountability…

…which enables the worker either to engage in collusive alliances or to avoid engagement with others – both of which support the 'stuck' position…

…which reduces feedback from others about the impact of one's behaviour, or personal awareness of dangerous emotions…

…which makes the worker's role manageable and predictable and reduces exposure to new situations and uncertainty…

…which enables the worker to regain a sense of safety, predictability and competence.

Adapted from Morrison T (2005)

In this way under-performance, while professionally and publicly problematic, is privately functional as a self-protective response to anxiety, uncertainty and unpredictability. It is important to note that this is not an argument for ignoring or colluding with under-performance. Instead, the blocked cycle offers a more comprehensive way of understanding what might be causing the blocked behaviour.

It also points to the fact that strategies for dealing with under-performance require accurate information, high quality feedback and a containing and authoritative approach if they are to successfully 'unblock' the social worker. The following strategies may need to be considered once the nature of the block has been identified.

Strategies when the worker is stuck in reflection

■ Clarify the worker's understanding of the task.

■ Make clear your expectations about what has to be done.

■ Check what skills, knowledge and experience the worker needs to do the task. Identify any training needs.

■ Ask the worker how the task is similar to something else they have managed previously.

■ Explore what happened when the worker performed a similar task; identify the positive and negative outcomes. Check whether these were related to issues of race, gender etc.

■ Break the task down into manageable parts that are within the worker's own perception of competence, and prioritise what needs to be done.

■ Check out what the worker's worst fear or fantasy is about what could happen.

■ Give feedback pointing out the worker's strengths and experience.

■ Identify processes which may be unhelpful or disempowering to the worker in the way s/he is either thinking or behaving.

■ Suggest colleagues who can share some of the task or co-work.

■ Offer the chance to observe an experienced worker doing the task.

■ Set time limits on getting things done, specifying how the work is to be recorded.

- Ensure your availability to see the worker soon after they have done the task.

- Ask the worker to specify the help s/he wants from you or anyone else.

- Arrange a rehearsal of the task.

- Ask the worker how s/he will feel once the task is completed.

- After completing the task, help the worker analyse what they did well, and areas for further work.

Pitfall

Do not focus too much on feelings. This is where the worker is stuck!

Strategies where the worker is stuck in analysis

- Check out what feelings the worker has around the task.

- Note and give feedback if questions about feelings are answered with thoughts, theoretical response or generalisations. This may have a gender-mediate element.

- Pursue 'feelings' answers to 'feelings' questions.

- Ask the worker to undertake a process record of a task in order to raise their awareness of the experience they are engaged in.

- Check out what fears or fantasies the worker has about doing the task and whether these are related to factors of race, gender etc.

- Maintain focus on the issue and avoid being drawn into generalisations or intellectualisation.

- Acknowledge the validity of different theoretical/political perspectives but point out agency, ethical or legal obligations to the task or user.

- Schedule other times to discuss these more general issues which are of concern to the worker.

- Clarify the exact nature of the task, break it down and prioritise what needs to be done when. Set a review date.

- Identify what help the worker would like to complete the task.

- Set up rehearsal opportunities.

- Identify training needs.

- Check whether being stuck like this is familiar to the worker. It may be rooted in an earlier bad experience, or in a more fundamental realisation that the nature of the job is in conflict with moral or political convictions. If so, offer time to review the worker's career options and aspirations.

Pitfall

Avoid entanglement or competition over intellectual debates.

Strategies when the worker is stuck in action

- Ensure full attendance at supervision sessions.

- Check out how the worker is feeling about his/her work and the pressures of the job.

- Be prepared for considerable defensiveness. The worker may fear any examination of his/her worker is an attempt to invalidate all the hours they have put in. The 'busy-ness' may be masking personal needs, and require sensitive handling.

- Recognise the worker's commitment and abilities.

- Identify examples of good work and use them to help the worker compare these with less competent work in order to highlight areas for change.

- Find a positive rationale for the changes which you are seeking; for example, you are concerned about working too hard, or that the worker's skills can be used more productively.

- Ask the worker to summarise plans, goals and rationale for involvement in a particular case. Avoid long anecdotes about what the worker has done. Request written summaries with case plans for cases.

- Check the condition and whereabouts of the case files.

- Identify training or re-training needs.

- Analyse the worker's time management. This should include a look at his/her agency diary. It is agency not personal time that the worker is managing.

- Clarify expectations about accountability and reporting arrangements to you.

- Consider whether there are any needs for counselling and, if so, how the agency should support such a need.

- Assess whether they can, with help, continue to do the current job. If not, explore within the agency other options.

Pitfall

Ensure that, while being sensitive, you maintain a clear boundary as supervisor and do not become drawn into being friend, counsellor or rescuer.

Strategies when the worker is stuck in experience

(a) Where some form of burnout is suspected

- Seek information about the symptoms of burnout.

- Check sickness and lateness records.

- Ascertain how the worker is feeling about work, levels of satisfaction, dissatisfaction, sense of progress, future hopes and aspirations. Be prepared for denial or anger.

- Review worker's caseload and commitments. Are they excessive?

- Identify training or re-training needs.

- Clarify that the worker is clear as to roles and responsibilities.

- Sensitively check out if there is anything else going on in the worker's life which may account for his/her presentation.

- Audit files and performance carefully. Someone who is burnt out will be very desensitised to areas of risk, needs and distress with users. Check that the worker's accounts are accurate.

- Give specific feedback about attitudes and behaviour you have observed which have made you suspect burnout.

- Discuss the issues with your supervisor/personnel department and consider the need to seek a medical opinion. There can be important but hidden physiological signs associated with burnout which will require medical help. A medical examination is a staff care intervention and can help the worker to see what is happening. A significant rest from work may be required.

■ In the light of all the above, review with the worker the ability to continue in the current post, either temporarily or in the long term. Prepare possible options in consultation with your manager/personnel department.

Pitfall

Be careful not to be so concerned about the staff care aspect in dealing with burnout that accountability issues are neglected.

(b) Where the worker appears to be frozen or immobilised
(Many of the strategies for those who are stuck in reflection also apply here.)

■ Clarify the worker's perception of the role and responsibilities.

■ Clarify the worker's expectations as to skill, knowledge and experience.

■ These may be inflated and unrealistic.

■ Check out in detail the worker's training and developmental needs.

■ Identify what the worker feels confident about.

■ Check out whether there has been a specific incident or event that has caused distress or loss of confidence.

■ Discuss how you will provide constructive feedback and ask how the worker can best use supervision to build confidence.

■ Discuss how you will provide constructive feedback and ask how the worker can best use supervision to build confidence.

■ Negotiate gradual build-up of responsibility with regular review points. There can be a tension between the worker's wish to return to work and your judgement about whether the worker is ready.

■ Check out previous agency and supervisory history. Is there anything unresolved that is 'blocking' the worker? Pay particular attention to experiences of discrimination or previous incidents of distress which were insensitively handled.

- Explore the worker's understanding of the work, the agency and the decision to join your team. Is the worker sure this is the right job or post?

Note: It will be important not to exclude the possibility of this being the initial stages of burnout and therefore some of the strategies mentioned above may be relevant. However, the worker here is more likely to be fearful or diffident than cynical and negative. There may not be any obvious precipitating incident.

Pitfall

Don't assume that because you have reassured the worker of their ability to do the job that the worker can internalise your positive feedback ie. is able to believe you!

Improving performance through positive reinforcement

The positive reinforcement approach, which is based on social learning theory, states that behaviour that is positively rewarded is more likely to be repeated or maintained. Positive reinforcement includes both social rewards such as thanks, praise or recognition of work well done, as well as tangible rewards such as developmental opportunities, career progression or role expansion.

Using a positive reinforcement approach in situations where there are performance concerns involves:

- accurate observation of the worker's performance

- assessment and analysis of the worker's performance including concerns

- self-assessment of the supervisor's performance

- knowledge of organisational and professional policies and standards

- feedback about performance concerns that is based on clear evidence

- explanation of why the supervisor is concerned and the required standards

- discussion to gain a shared understanding of the reasons for the problem

- careful goal-setting: clarifying what needs to change, and what improved performance would look like

- developmental, work-redesign or occupational health strategies to enable improvements

- regular and, if necessary, enhanced supervision

- clear documentation of the above

- careful reviewing of progress and clarification of next steps if there has been no improvement.

Giving feedback

Morrison (2005) identifies that giving and receiving constructive feedback on a regular basis are two of the most powerful but under-used tools available for improving performance. Unfortunately, one of the reasons it is under-used is that some staff and supervisors have had such bad experiences that they no longer regard it as a useful or safe tool. Nonetheless, all staff at all levels of the organisation deserve and need regular feedback to work at their best.

Giving feedback works best when it is:

- **Planned:** Prepare what you need to say carefully. A muddled delivery will result in a rapid escalation of anxiety and misunderstanding. Think about the timing and location, too. Consider how the worker might respond. Has he or she had prior negative experiences of feedback? What might the worker's supervision history suggest?

- **Clear and owned:** 'I want to give you some feedback about how I saw you dealing with that meeting.'

- **Soon:** Do not leave it so long after the event such that the worker feels they can no longer rectify the situation.

- **Balanced:** Feed back that it highlights both strengths and weaknesses, though not necessarily at the same time. You do not want the worker to associate positive feedback as a prelude to criticism.

- **Specific and behaviour-focused:** A worker cannot change their personality but can change their behaviour. The biggest problem with feedback is that it is too often non-specific.

Whatever strategies supervisors use to improve performance, they need to work within a context which supports them in this task. Morrison (2005) identified a number of building blocks that need to be in place for supervisors and any gaps need to be identified before any complex issues arise. For example, if no agreement is in place outlining roles and expectations, challenges to practice performance may be viewed negatively and even seen as oppressive or bullying. Supervisors lacking emotional support within their own supervisory relationships may avoid difficult conversations or become overwhelmed and this is particularly likely when they are lacking clear HR support and advice.

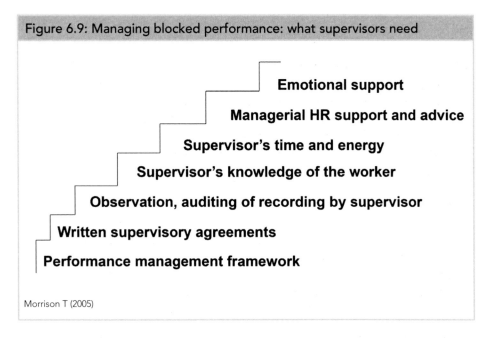

Figure 6.9: Managing blocked performance: what supervisors need

Emotional support

Managerial HR support and advice

Supervisor's time and energy

Supervisor's knowledge of the worker

Observation, auditing of recording by supervisor

Written supervisory agreements

Performance management framework

Morrison T (2005)

Further issues relating to the support and development of supervisors are discussed in the concluding chapter.

References

Carpenter J, Webb C, Bostock L & Coomber C (2012) *Effective Supervision in Social Work and Social Care*. London: SCIE.

Cooperrider DL, Whitney D & Stavros JM (2008) *Appreciative Inquiry Handbook*. Ohio: Crown Custom Publishing.

Hughes L & Pengelly P (1997) *Staff Supervision in a Turbulent World*. London: Jessica Kingsley.

Lambley S & Marrable T (2013) *Practice Enquiry into Supervision in a Variety of Adult Care Settings where there are Health and Social Care Practitioners Working Together*. London: SCIE.

Manzoni J-F & Barsoux J-L (1999) 'The Set-Up-to-Fail Syndrome' in *Harvard Business Review on Managing People*. Harvard Business School Press.

Morrison T (2005) *Staff Supervision in Social Care*. Brighton: Pavilion.

Rogers S (1999) *Performance Management in Local Government* (2nd edition) Chapter 7 'The management of individual performance' pp113–148. London: Financial Times/Pitman London.

Vroom V (1964) *Work and Motivation*. New York, NY: Wiley.

Wonnacott J (2012) *Mastering Social Work Supervision*. London: JKP.

Chapter 7:
Supervision training in context: supporting, developing and sustaining supervisors

This reader accompanies a training manual designed to address some of the core training needs of supervisors working in health, social care or similar environments and sets out ideas for various short training programmes. However, supervisors need far more than a short training course and this chapter explores the context within which training needs to take place and additional support mechanisms for maximising the impact of training on supervisory practice across the organisation.

Training is likely to have most impact when strategies to support and develop supervisors are operating at the level of the organisation, peer group and individual.

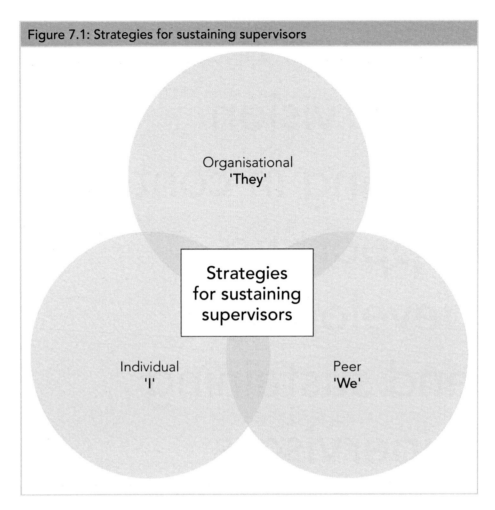

Figure 7.1: Strategies for sustaining supervisors

- *Organisational* strategies include the development of an effective supervision culture, high quality supervision for supervisors and regular observation and feedback on the day-to-day practice of supervision.

- *Peer* strategies may include action learning opportunities.

- *Individual* strategies include developing self-awareness and capacity to seek help.

The role of the organisation in sustaining and supporting supervisors

Morrison (2005) identified organisational building blocks for effective supervision; training for supervisors is just one small element within the whole system and any organisation that relies solely on training to deliver effective supervision is bound to fail.

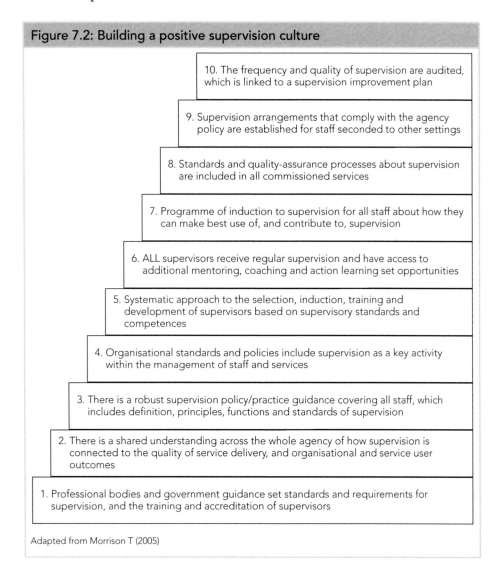

Figure 7.2: Building a positive supervision culture

10. The frequency and quality of supervision are audited, which is linked to a supervision improvement plan

9. Supervision arrangements that comply with the agency policy are established for staff seconded to other settings

8. Standards and quality-assurance processes about supervision are included in all commissioned services

7. Programme of induction to supervision for all staff about how they can make best use of, and contribute to, supervision

6. ALL supervisors receive regular supervision and have access to additional mentoring, coaching and action learning set opportunities

5. Systematic approach to the selection, induction, training and development of supervisors based on supervisory standards and competences

4. Organisational standards and policies include supervision as a key activity within the management of staff and services

3. There is a robust supervision policy/practice guidance covering all staff, which includes definition, principles, functions and standards of supervision

2. There is a shared understanding across the whole agency of how supervision is connected to the quality of service delivery, and organisational and service user outcomes

1. Professional bodies and government guidance set standards and requirements for supervision, and the training and accreditation of supervisors

Adapted from Morrison T (2005)

Who are the supervisors? A whole system approach to developing supervision practice

As shown by **Figure 6.1**, supervision does not take place in isolation and is likely to work best where senior managers recognise the connections between organisational goals, service delivery, service user outcomes and the quality of supervision. This does, however, need to move beyond a linear understanding of impact, to a whole systems approach which addresses the question of who are the supervisors. Unless an organisation moves beyond seeing reflective-style supervision as solely the province of those supervising frontline staff, and unless senior managers recognise that they are supervisors too, it is unlikely that effective supervision will be sustained over time.

Unfortunately many supervisors report that they do not receive the style of supervision that they are required to give. Lawson, for example, notes:

'When I have asked first-line supervisors about their own supervision, it becomes clear that for the majority their own supervision is inadequate. It is often described as overly task-focused and a "quick check-in".' (Community Care, 2011)

This is despite the fact that many supervisors are working in situations of high stress and anxiety. For example, a survey of managers across public and private sectors concluded that it was the frontline managers in the public sector who experienced the largest amount of organisational change and reported the greatest degree of stress. The research concluded that although accountability had improved, this was often at the cost of 'dramatic decreases of managers' loyalty, morale, motivation and job security' (Worrall *et al*, 2001).

Under-confident, untrained and unsupported supervisors are poorly placed to offer their staff what they need to practise well. In order to sustain effective supervision beyond an initial flush of enthusiasm gained on a training course, supervisors need high quality supervision themselves, as well as other learning and development opportunities.

Lawson, however, points out that the situation is more complicated than simply senior managers being unable or unwilling to offer effective supervision. She notes:

'Many first-line supervisors begin to reveal that it is they who avoid long sessions with their supervisor because they assume they won't get their needs met or because they feel unsure in their role and don't want the risk of exposure or because to need supervision is equated with 'not being able to cope'. It seems as though once a practitioner has moved away from the front line, seeking support and supervision is tantamount to admitting failure.'
(Ofsted, 2012)

It is here we see the importance of the fit between the quality of supervision and the overall culture of the organisation; a culture that will to a large extent be determined by those in leadership roles and played out in the way that they manage and supervise others. If supervisors are, as Lawson (2011) suggests, fearful of the consequences of seeking support this establishes even more clearly the need to pay attention to the overall culture within which supervision is delivered.

Supervisors have described themselves as feeling like the jam in the sandwich squeezed from both sides by demands from the organisation and their supervisees without attention being paid to the emotional impact of the work on them. One danger of this is that the supervisor will retreat into defensive behaviour. Such behaviour may be similar to that described by Menzies-Lyth (1970) who studied the high level of stress and anxiety exhibited by nurses and understood this in terms of the need to defend against intolerable anxiety through, amongst other things, the depersonalisation of the individual. Supervisors who do not receive the support they need may therefore distance themselves from their supervisees and fail to engage with each person as an individual with very different needs and circumstances. Distancing behaviour may result in lack of focus on the detail of the work, particularly the emotional demands and complex relationships and failure to challenge poor practice. Alternatively, supervisors may protect themselves through collusive behaviour with their supervisees with the belief that they are protecting them from the demands of the organisation. Poor performance is not challenged, therefore the demands of the organisation increase and pressure is exerted on the supervisor to improve practice and a negative cycle is set up.

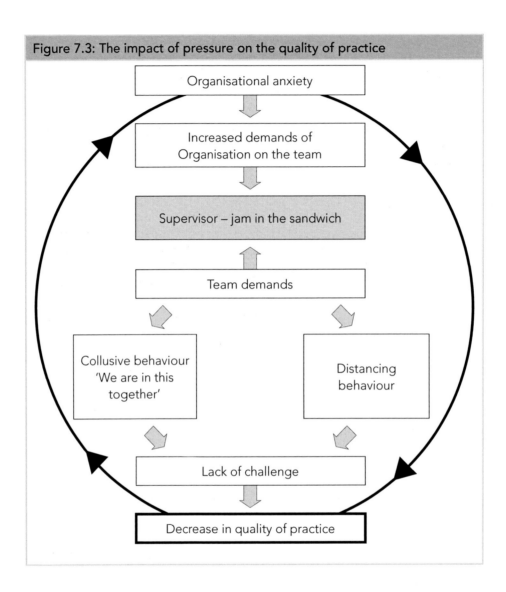

Figure 7.3: The impact of pressure on the quality of practice

Preventing this negative cycle therefore depends on supervisors getting good supervision themselves. This needs to be part of a whole system approach to the delivery of supervision, within which the needs of even the most senior managers for reflective space and emotional support are understood as a vital component in the development of the critical thinking required for them to be effective in their role.

Observation and supervisee feedback

The quality of supervision needs to be regularly monitored, yet research by Ofsted (2012) noted that only a minority of social workers and managers stated that this happened. One of the most influential ways in which an organisation can monitor supervision and influence quality is by making conversations about supervision practice 'ordinary'. Two ways of doing this are through regular feedback from supervisees and observation of supervision sessions.

Supervisee feedback can be obtained via questionnaires and surveys, but one of the most powerful ways is a structured observation of a supervision session at the end of which supervisor, supervisee and observer engage in a reflective discussion about the supervision process. These observations can be carried out by an external facilitator but are arguably most useful if undertaken internally and used to inform the overall development of supervision practice within the organisation. However, where this is built into the system there are number of important considerations.

- Does the observer have a good understanding of what good supervision looks like?

- Have they been trained in the same model of supervision being used by the supervisor?

- Does the supervisee have a good understanding of what good supervision looks like?

- Have they had training in what to expect from supervision and the model of supervision being used within the organisation?

- Are the boundaries for the observation negotiated and clear? For example, confidentiality and its limits, and the use and storage of any records kept by the observer?

- Are the 'rules' for the observation process clear? For example, are there any instances when the observer might intervene, who will feedback first following the session? Good practice would generally dictate that the supervisor should always have first opportunity to comment on how the session went from their perspective as they are the person most likely to feel 'on the spot', followed by the supervisee and lastly the observer.

Developing and using peer support

Much of what is required to put supervisors on a firm footing has been described within in the organisational building blocks explored above. However, negotiating tough times, difficult team processes, tricky personalities, and hard decisions can undermine the supervisor's ability, knowledge, judgement, confidence, and authority. Under such pressures, the very identity of the supervisor comes into question as he/she begins to wonder exactly who they are.

Morrison, in unpublished training materials, refers to this as the supervisor's balancing act.

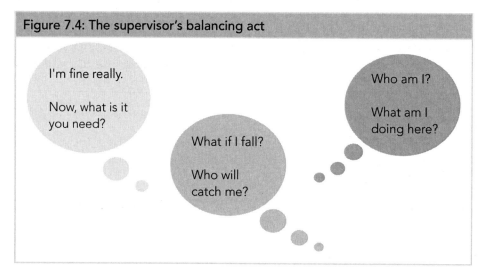

Figure 7.4: The supervisor's balancing act

I'm fine really.

Now, what is it you need?

What if I fall?

Who will catch me?

Who am I?

What am I doing here?

It is when supervisors are faced with profound challenges and doubts about their efficacy, peer support is of greatest value in providing a safe space for reflection. While elements of this can happen in a number of ways, ranging from informal social support to buddying and mentoring, Morrison (2010), exploring the strategic leadership of frontline practice, argues that supervisors need a structured space where they can reduce their isolation and:

- feel safe enough to acknowledge their true feeling

- recognise uncertainty and doubt as a powerful aid

- get connected to and engaged with other supervisors

- tell it like it is (not how the organisation would like it to be)

- share knowledge, information and know-how
- contribute to the solution of others' problems
- regain a sense of collective value and competence as supervisors
- recharge their batteries and refocus their energies.

One of the most effective and comprehensive structures for peer support is action learning sets.

Action learning sets

Revans (1982), who created the idea of action learning sets, described them as the 'development of the self by the mutual support of equals'. These are structured opportunities for a group of supervisors to work together on common problems over a period of time. As the term suggests, they are about learning through action. In other words, good action learning sets go beyond professional support and development to address the members' needs for a secure, or at least secure enough, sense of self and identity in their roles. As Payne (2006) states, we cannot construct or maintain an identity unless we participate in action with others.

The basic principles of action learning sets (Mumford, 1991) are:

- learning involves actually taking action, not just talking about it
- action involves work on a project/problem that is significant for the supervision
- learning is a social process
- the social process is carried out through group meetings
- groups are helped to learn by exposure to problems and each other
- there is a facilitator.

According to Morrison (in unpublished training materials), in facilitating action learning sets for supervisors, a common process seems to occur that involves re-connecting and engaging, followed by a process of sharing feelings and 'telling it like it is'. The importance of hearing each other and acknowledging each other's collective realities cannot be over-emphasised, even when this means hearing about sometimes impossible demands, irresolvable problems, and unrelenting pressures along with the doubt, worry, and anger or despair that can accompany such situations.

However, this stage of 'hitting the bottom' is often followed by a reverse thrust in which members spontaneously start to identify exceptions when things have worked, which generates alternative stories and possibilities. Simply inviting supervisors to identify just one thing that has worked (despite all the mayhem around them) and how they have contributed to this, is often enough to puncture the 'nothing works' atmosphere.

From there, the process moves to working on an identified issue. Sometimes this can be generated by members or it may be an issue for which the organisation has sought the help of the set. Reciprocity in helping relationships is one of the keys to recovering a sense of competence, as supervisors move from being help-seekers to help-givers. Developing commitments to take action on issues and partners with whom to work is essential as we learn by doing, and it is through taking action that our identity is consolidated. Finally, the set takes time to reflect on their learning with particular reference to the process by which the group has worked together and what this tells members about who they are and who they can be.

Supervisors in action learning sets frequently comment on the uniqueness and importance of a safe space in the organisation, to share feelings, worries and doubts where their basic humanity can be recognised. Good action learning sets create a culture of possibility and capability, but above all, action learning sets restore morale.

Individual strategies

Ultimately, however good the organisational and peer support processes, the supervisor chooses whether and how to use them. The factors that affect the use that supervisees make of supervision will also affect supervisors themselves.

Commenting on the personal responsibility that all workers have in the face of work-related stress, Morrison (2005) argues:

'... this should not be taken to imply that individuals do not have personal responsibilities in the face of work related stress – they do. Indeed the demands of today's working environment suggest that individual robustness and emotional competence are increasingly important and should be a *focus during recruitment and selection. Individuals who show little sense of personal responsibility, for whom problems are always the agency's fault, are more likely to succumb under pressure. At the opposite end, workers who take too much personal responsibility are equally vulnerable. Therefore, realistic attitudes and the use of positive coping strategies are very important.*

Developing the capacity to bounce back in the face of adversity and cope with life's challenges has been extensively explored in relation to service users within the resilience literature (Newman, 2004). More recently this has been researched within the work environment and its importance explored for the individual in protecting their own well-being and enhancing professional practice. Research into social work suggests that resilient social workers are those who:

'are able to maintain positive relationships, access support from a range of sources, demonstrate appropriate empathy, draw on a range of coping styles and successfully manage and contain their own emotions and those of others. More resilient social workers are able to reflect constructively on their practice, set firm physical and emotional boundaries between home and work domains, and derive a sense of meaning from the challenges they face.' (Grant, 2012)

Individual capacity for resilience will be affected by combinations of environmental and individual factors but it the most resilient workers and supervisors who will be most likely to access the support systems available to them. In order to help supervisors reflect on their own capacity for resilience, Morrison (2005) set out a self-awareness checklist to assist supervisors in identifying their resilience skills and strengths.

Developing a secure identity as a supervisor

Help-seeking behaviour is likely to be affected by the degree to which the individual feels secure in their identity as a supervisor and is also able to maintain this under pressure when they might be most vulnerable and in need of support. For example, the supervisor who is uncertain of who they are in their role might be more likely to feel that help-seeking behaviour is a sign of weakness. Supervisors will develop their identity within the role over time, yet all too often the distinction between role (what I do) and identity (who I am) is not recognised, particularly in the early stages of their supervisory development.

This is where training courses can help with supervisors having the opportunity to develop confidence in their role. Through reflecting on their own history of being supervised and working with peers they can try on the role, discover themselves as a supervisor and reflect on how they wish to be in the role. Continuation of this process through action learning and their own supervision will be equally important.

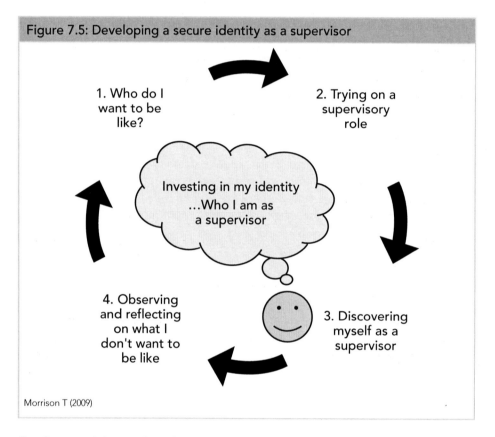

Figure 7.5: Developing a secure identity as a supervisor

1. Who do I want to be like?

2. Trying on a supervisory role

Investing in my identity ...Who I am as a supervisor

4. Observing and reflecting on what I don't want to be like

3. Discovering myself as a supervisor

Morrison T (2009)

Good supervision and positive outcomes for service users are inextricably bound together and ultimately developing, supporting and sustaining supervisors is one of the most important tasks of any human services organisation. The message from this reader is that training is only one aspect of this process and the most successful organisations are likely to be those where all supervisors receive the same high quality supervision they are expected to deliver, have regular development opportunities including peer support and are regularly challenged to reflect on their practice through observation and supervisee feedback. All organisations should have high expectations of their supervisors but equally need to reflect on the way in which the whole system can work together to maximise the likelihood of success.

References

Community Care (2011) 'Inform' 21/4/11 (electronic; subscribers only).

Grant L (2012) Guide to developing social worker emotional resilience. *Community Care* 'Inform' 4/7/11 (electronic; subscribers only).

Lawson H (2011) Guide to effective supervision: what is it and how can supervisors ensure they provide it?' *Community Care* 'Inform' 21/4/11 (electronic; subscribers only).

Menzies-Lyth L (1970) *The Functioning of Social Systems as a Defence Against Anxiety*. London: Tavistock Institute of Human Relations.

Morrison T (2005) *Staff Supervision in Social Care*. Brighton: Pavilion.

Morrison T (2009) Unpublished training materials.

Morrison T (2010) The strategic leadership of complex practice. *Child Abuse Review* **19** 312–329.

Mumford A (1991) Individual and organizational learning – the pursuit of change. *Industrial and Commercial Training* **23** (6).

Newman T (2004) *What Works in Building Resilience*. London: Barnardos.

Ofsted (2012) *High Expectation, High Support and High Challenge: Protecting children more effectively through frontline social work practice* No. 110120. Available at: http://dera.ioe.ac.uk/13875/ (accessed October 2013).

Payne M (2006) Identity politics in multi-professional teams. *Journal of Social Work* **6** (2) pp137–150.

Revans R (1982) *The Origins and Growth of Action Learning*. Chartwell-Bratt: Bromley UK.

Worrall L, Cooper C & Campbell F (2001) The pathology of organisational change: a study of UK managers' experiences. In: B Hamblin, J Keep and K Ask (eds) *Organisational Change and Development*. Harlow: Financial Times/Prentice Hall.